M000014911

SO YOU WANT TO BE A VETERINARIAN

What Every Aspiring DVM Should Know

Robert F. Kahrs, DVM, PhD

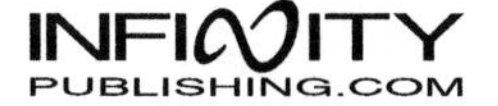

First Published as an Infinity Paperback by Robert F. Kahrs
bobkahrs@aol.com
Library of Congress Cataloging-in-Publication Data
Kahrs, Robert, F.
So You Want to Be a Veterinarian
ISBN 0-7414-5623-0
1. Veterinary Medicine. 2. Veterinary College Admissions.
3. Veterinary Careers

Published by:

INFINITY
PUBLISHING.COM

1094 New DeHaven Street, Suite 100
West Conshohocken, PA 19428-2713
Info@buybooksontheweb.com
www.buybooksontheweb.com
Toll-free (877) BUY BOOK
Local Phone (610) 941-9999
Fax (610) 941-9959

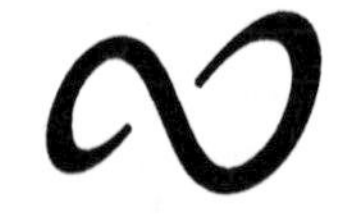

Printed in the United States of America

Published September 2009

CONTENTS

ABOUT THE COVERS

The front cover of this book contains photos of real-life veterinary activities.

In the upper left is Jack Lowe, DVM, MS, a 1959 graduate of Cornell University and Professor Emeritus of Population Medicine and Diagnostic Services at Cornell. He is examining the suspensory ligament and flexor tendons of a Dutch Warmblood horse at the New Jersey State Fair in 2009.

In the upper right is Anne Payne Fessler, DVM, a 1980 graduate of Cornell University. She is a private practitioner. In the photo, she is examining the eye of a dog in her clinic in Farmington, New York. The photo was taken in 2009.

In the lower left is Judy Lincoln. She is Volunteer Facilities Coordinator for the University of Missouri's veterinary student-operated Raptor Rehabilitation Project. She is holding Willie the hawk. Willie was brought to the veterinary college by the Missouri Conservation Department in 1995, and veterinary students have cared for him ever since. He has multiple wing injuries that limit his ability to fly. Students care for many other injured birds, which are released when their health returns to normal. The photo was taken in 2008.

In the lower right is Carlos Risco, DVM, a 1980 graduate of the University of Florida (UFL), where he is a professor of dairy medicine. In the photo, he is conducting a herd health visit and examining a chopped mixed ration for milking cows at the UFL College of Agriculture's dairy farm in 2008.

On the back cover is the author's photo. It was taken in 2008 by Lyn LaBar of the Cornell University College of Veterinary Medicine, Office of Alumni Affairs.

FOREWORD

In this concise book, Dr. Robert Kahrs, former dean of the College of Veterinary Medicine at the University of Missouri, addresses a wide range of considerations of students and others considering this career path. Dr. Kahrs draws upon his extensive personal knowledge and vast years of experience to advise his readers.

The book is organized in 13 chapters, each addressing an important aspect of the veterinary profession which should be of interest to the reader. The book describes the profession and how it is organized, and lists and describes the accredited schools and colleges. There is an overview of the kinds of career opportunities available to veterinarians and the kinds of specialized fields within the profession. It also provides a glimpse of the kinds of courses and topics that are delivered in a veterinary college curriculum.

Finally Dr. Kahrs provides some advice and tips to prospective applicants on how to approach the admission process. He even gives advice to students on specific habits and behaviors that will enhance their study habits and academic performance. These are recommendations to live by.

I think this book gives a valuable glimpse into an exciting profession full of opportunities. Anyone interested in entering veterinary college should read this book.

Glen F. Hoffsis, DVM, Dean
College of Veterinary Medicine
University of Florida

PREFACE

Many young people consider becoming a veterinarian. With some, it is a passing fancy, but with many others it is a serious desire that becomes embedded at an early age and lingers quietly until they mention it to someone. Those with whom they share this wish may applaud and encourage them or judge and discourage them. This book strongly suggests encouragement. It lays out a logical pathway to success, which requires effort by potential applicants and support from their mentors and friends.

This book discusses veterinary medicine and the challenges involved in obtaining access to this well-respected profession. It is intended for potential applicants to colleges of veterinary medicine and also for their parents, siblings, relatives, teachers, coaches, scoutmasters, and mentors of all kinds.

So You Want to Be a Veterinarian describes the veterinary profession and lists each veterinary college in the US and Canada. It discusses the variable admission requirements and curriculums. It offers suggestions for youth of all ages on how to begin preparing for the challenges of applying to veterinary colleges and outlines the application procedures. It also describes the careers open to veterinary graduates, some animal health organizations, and the challenges facing the profession.

It discusses some realities and challenges facing applicants to veterinary colleges and indicates that admission is possible for those who are determined and willing to work at it.

Many people provided the experiences and inspirations that led to this book. I am grateful to my parents and many mentors through high school and college. They pointed me in directions that permitted a veterinary education. I also thank the many colleagues in practice, academe, and government who guided and supported me in multiple veterinary careers and provided the background and perspectives needed to finalize this manuscript.

I thank my granddaughter Kierston Kahrs for designing the cover, and Beth Mansbridge, my wife Evelyn, Dr. Glen Hoffsis, and Cindy Kahrs (my daughter) for editing, and I thank Cindy and her husband, Kelly, for installing the new computer.

Most of all, I thank Evelyn for her patience, love, and support in my lifelong efforts to master writing and to succeed in this wonderful profession.

INTRODUCTION

If you, one of your friends, one of your children, or one of your students, want to be a veterinarian, this book will help. It describes a rewarding career that requires careful planning, dedicated preparation, and hard work. Becoming a veterinarian is a challenging goal. Careers requiring less education are available as veterinary assistants, veterinary technicians, and veterinary technologists.

Many people think all that veterinarians do is neuter cats and dogs and treat sick or injured pets. Beyond that, few individuals have knowledge of the career opportunities, lifestyles, and earning capacities of veterinarians.

So You Want to Be a Veterinarian offers suggestions for aspiring doctors of veterinary medicine and those who support them. It addresses common perceptions about veterinary medicine and offers strategies for pursuing the Doctor of Veterinary Medicine (DVM) degree. This book describes the veterinary medical profession and the many career choices open to recipients of veterinary degrees.

If possible, preparation for veterinary careers should begin in grade school and expand throughout middle school, high school, and college. The approaches described are applicable to many careers and professions.

This Book

So You Want to Be a Veterinarian: What Every Aspiring DVM Should Know describes the various facets of the veterinary profession and the varied practice opportunities that are available.

It also details many unheralded—but extremely rewarding —non-practice veterinary careers and the contributions veterinarians make to society while employed in academic, corporate, and governmental organizations.

So You Want to Be a Veterinarian encourages and supports potential applicants to veterinary colleges and offers positive suggestions for their mentors. Chapters one through six discuss the veterinary profession, colleges of veterinary medicine, preparation for application, the application process, and veterinary college curriculums in general terms that may be understood by interested students of all ages. Chapters seven through twelve outline veterinary careers, veterinary specialties, veterinary organizations, and the challenges facing the veterinary profession. They can be skimmed until readers encounter an area of their particular interest and wish more detail.

This book urges potential applicants to realistically address the challenges of admission to veterinary colleges. It suggests that all aspiring veterinarians undertake academic, extra-curricular, and community activities as early as possible. These endeavors will help potential veterinarians develop attitudes and habits that will serve for a lifetime and expedite the achievement of many career goals.

CHAPTER 1

THE VETERINARY PROFESSION

Introduction

Veterinary medicine is an unusual and highly respected profession with many dimensions that are unknown to the general public. Most US veterinarians have six to ten years of college education before receiving a Doctor of Veterinary Medicine (DVM) or Veterinary Medical Doctor (VMD) degree. Many serve additional years in internships, residencies, or graduate programs as they train for specialties.

After selecting a veterinary career, veterinarians usually spend productive and rewarding lives as well-respected professionals and often assume leadership positions in their communities.

The Character of the Profession

About half of US and Canadian veterinarians are engaged in private practice. Veterinarians classified as practitioners conduct small animal, large animal, or mixed practices, and many have species or discipline specialty practices. While working in clinics, animal hospitals, and laboratories, many veterinarians supervise employees and manage organizational and business operations.

Some who are involved in teaching or research often have MS or PhD degrees in addition to the DVM. These long and intense educational programs require unique talents, abilities, and patience. After graduation, many veterinary skills must be perfected by hands-on experience.

Academic, corporate, and government veterinarians conduct a variety of professional and regulatory activities involving teaching, research, animal health, public health, food safety, and oversight of animal experimentation. Veterinarians are employed by universities, pharmaceutical companies, and governmental agencies including the military. In all settings, veterinarians working directly with animals are considered clinicians. Others who may not work directly with animals are often called basic scientists, regulatory veterinarians, or corporate veterinarians.

Veterinarians often enter non-practice phases of the profession after a stint in practice because they develop increased enthusiasm for certain specialties or become restless, exhausted, or disabled. People are largely unaware of the vastness of veterinary activities because most people's contact with veterinarians is largely limited to the treatment of privately owned animals. Most US veterinary practices involve companion animals (dogs and cats). The others are divided among practices handling farm animals, horses, poultry, pet birds, laboratory animals, aquatic animals, or zoo animals.

The financial rewards of veterinary medicine are modest compared to human medicine, computer technology, and business leadership. Only a few veterinarians get very wealthy, but most make comfortable livings and have desirable lifestyles. Some that have exceptional drive achieve great wealth.

Veterinary Technologists, Technicians, and Assistants

Over the years many veterinarians have had helpers who assisted them with a variety of chores. Frequently, companion animal veterinarians hire assistants to answer phones, care for animals, clean kennels, and perform essential duties in their clinics. Large animal practitioners often have helpers to carry their equipment, restock their vehicles, restrain animals, run errands, and sometimes drive their cars.

As these assistants gain experience and earn the confidence of their employers, they are usually introduced to more complicated tasks like determining the temperature, pulse and respiratory rates of animals, using stethoscopes, performing vaccinations, and administering medications and injections. Large animal practitioners sometimes teach assistants to perform pregnancy examinations, deliver calves, and dehorn cattle. Practitioners rarely let assistants perform these services in their absence.

If something goes wrong, the veterinarian has to accept the responsibility and can possibly be accused of malpractice. In the past, a few veterinary assistants started their own business in direct competition with their former employers and other area veterinarians. This amounted to practicing veterinary medicine without the required training or license. Although such abuses were rare, the situation required attention, and formal veterinary technician training programs emerged.

Some individuals or groups distinguish among the levels of technician training, skills, and educational backgrounds. An unofficial classification emerged designating three levels of expertise, namely: veterinary assistants, veterinary technicians, and veterinary technologists.

In this nomenclature, high school graduates without further formal education are called assistants. Their tasks are limited to nonmedical procedures such as the care and housing of animals.

A second level is the veterinary technician with two years of post–high-school education in veterinary technology in a community college, junior college, or a veterinary technician program at a university. Technicians can be involved in patient care which can include taking temperatures and administering medications.

The third level—veterinary technologists—are graduates of four-year programs accredited by the American Veterinary Medical Association (AVMA). Veterinary technologists are qualified to undertake diagnostic and testing procedures and to operate diagnostic and therapeutic equipment under the direct supervision of veterinarians.

The AVMA has recognized the value of trained and well-supervised technicians and technologists, but has not emphasized the nomenclature described above. The AVMA has a program for accrediting the educational and training programs for veterinary technicians and technologists and for accrediting programs based on the training and skills of their graduates.

Most states oversee veterinary technicians and technologists by requiring that they be licensed, registered, or certified, and that they work directly with licensed veterinarians. These vocations offer alternatives to the prolonged training required for the Doctor of Veterinary Medicine (DVM) degree and they provide satisfying careers for individuals who choose to work with animals but are reluctant to pursue the prolonged educational requirements of the DVM degree.

Veterinary technicians and technologists are educated and trained in the care and handling of animals, in routine clinical procedures, and in some laboratory testing methods. They are usually prohibited by state laws from diagnosing diseases, prescribing medications, or performing surgery. They can prepare animals and instruments for surgery, assist veterinarians in surgery, and expose and develop X-rays.

In some states, technicians and technologists must take tests to get a license. In addition to working for practicing veterinarians, technicians and technologists assist veterinarians in diagnostic or research laboratories, colleges and universities, pharmaceutical companies, government and state agencies, and humane societies.

Veterinary technology is one option for individuals who desire regular working hours and who are comfortable being closely supervised yet are still interested in the handling and treatment of pets or livestock. It requires about a third of the education needed for the DVM degree and generates about a third of the income.

There are about 150 technician training programs approved by the AVMA Committee on Veterinary Technician Education and Activities. Of these, fewer than 20 are four-year-degree programs and about 10 of them offer distance learning programs accessible by computer.

Small Animal Practice

Most private practitioners deal mainly with dogs and cats. They are known as small animal practitioners. There is currently a movement toward a specialty (feline medicine), which deals exclusively with cats. However, most small animal practitioners treat both dogs and cats. Most will also address the problems of rabbits, birds, skunks, pet snakes, or other animals that show up in their offices.

Small animal veterinarians deal with the diagnosis, prevention, and treatment of illnesses and injuries, with routine vaccinations against infectious diseases, with surgical procedures, with a variety of routine illnesses—many of which present diagnostic challenges—and with emergency situations like traumatic injuries that occur when dogs or cats are hit by vehicles.

Small Animal Surgery

Elective surgeries for small animals involve spaying and neutering, tail docking, ear cropping, and de-clawing. Nonelective surgeries, those essential for survival or normal functioning, are performed to correct physical malfunctions such as swallowing of foreign objects that are capable of puncturing the gastrointestinal tract, repair of wounds and fractures, removal of tumors, or surgical correction of disorders of internal organs. All of these procedures are performed under local or general anesthesia.

Boarding and Grooming

Small animal practitioners often expand their operations by boarding and grooming pets. This permits a small animal clinic to offer a complete line of pet care.

Bathing and clipping in veterinary hospitals permits early recognition of parasite infestations and skin diseases which might otherwise be overlooked until they reach advanced stages. The income generated by boarding and grooming contributes to the maintenance and staffing of veterinary clinics.

Trends in Small Animal Practice

Ongoing trends in small animal practice include the replacement of solo practitioners (those who work alone) by group practices; establishment of animal emergency centers; a rapidly increasing number of women veterinarians; and the emergence of skilled specialists in small animal medicine and surgery.

Group Practices

Solo practices and two-doctor partnerships are being replaced by group practices owned by individuals or by multi-veterinarian corporations.

Group practices often hire recent graduates wishing to make the transition from college to the real world. The newcomers learn from their employers and in turn acquaint their mentors with the latest nuances from the colleges. Many stay with their original employers but most move on after a few years.

Animal Emergency Centers

Another small animal trend is establishment of animal emergency centers which are open all night and on holidays to accommodate urgent crises when many practices are closed. These are often operated by groups of practitioners who rotate nights and weekends so emergency service is always available. Participating practitioners usually resume responsibility for the pets of their regular clients during normal business hours.

Small Animal Clinical Specialties

As colleges of veterinary medicine adjusted to the increased emphasis on companion animal medicine, there emerged an increasing interest in small animal clinical specialties.

These specialties involve disciplines such as anesthesiology, animal behavior, cardiology, clinical pharmacology, dermatology, emergency medical services, endocrinology, internal medicine, neurology, radiology, reproduction, and surgery.

Most of these specialists were trained as interns, residents, or sometimes as graduate students with the goal of working as faculty at veterinary colleges. These specialists can attract clientele, sometimes from considerable distances, to provide teaching material for use by faculty and students.

As the numbers of clinical specialists expanded, they began leaving the academic community and establishing private specialty practices which competed with college clinics for referrals of challenging and unusual cases. This sometimes reduced the number of patients referred to veterinary college clinics.

Interest in small animal practice intensified, and there was a simultaneous reduction in the number of farms. The number of farm-reared applicants to veterinary colleges declined. This resulted in a shift in the interests of students and in the nature of the profession, producing a major turnaround of the profession by the beginning of the twenty-first century.

Large Animal Practice

Large animal practice includes horses and most food animal species. Poultry medicine, however, is a practice category of its own. Historically, veterinarians were called "horse doctors" (a term sometimes used disparagingly) since horses were once a major source of transportation. With the advent of autos, horse-powered equipment was largely limited to agricultural activities and by the 1900s food animal practice had emerged. When combined with equine practice, it was called large animal medicine.

In typical large animal practices, the veterinarian drives from farm to farm treating sick cattle, horses, sheep, goats, or swine; performing vaccinations; and developing and overseeing herd health programs. Large animal practitioners respond to emergencies such as problem births (dystocias) that require prompt expert treatment to save the mother and her offspring, and a variety of other potentially fatal disorders. Large animal practice requires 24-hour availability including weekends and holidays. It is exhausting and deprives participants of family time.

Large Animal Regulatory Programs

There are state or federally operated regulatory programs to control bovine brucellosis and tuberculosis, both of which can be transmitted to humans. Some of this work was formerly contracted out to large animal practitioners but is now largely performed by state and federal veterinarians.

Need for Large Animal Veterinarians

As small family farms were gradually being replaced by large corporate operations, the need for large animal practitioners appeared to be declining. However, other factors were at work. Traditionally, after 10 to 20 years of exhausting solo large animal practice, many large animal practitioners are ready for small animal practice or government or corporate employment where they can catch their breath on weekends and holidays. Initially these career-shifting veterinarians were easily replaced by recent graduates with interests in farm animal practice.

This worked well as long as young large animal veterinarians were eager to take over the clients. However, new graduates interested in large animal practice are no longer in abundant supply, so there is a shortage of food animal practitioners. Veterinary colleges are currently under pressure to provide coverage for food animal populations and are challenged both by a lack of interest and a shortage of students with farm backgrounds or agricultural interests. Many veterinary colleges are actively recruiting individuals interested in large animal practice.

This pattern may change if there is a rebirth of family-operated livestock farms. A similar transition is under way as new markets for locally grown fruit and vegetables are multiplying. Demand for locally produced meat and dairy products could also evolve, but currently there is little evidence of such a trend.

Mixed Practice

Many veterinary practitioners in rural areas meet the needs of all animal owners in their community and conduct what are known as mixed practices. Mixed practice provides a variety of experiences and there is never a dull moment.

Mixed practitioners are complete veterinarians and meet the needs of clientele with a wide variety of pets and livestock. They become known and respected in their communities and have a sense of belonging. They are always available and always busy. Mixed practitioners carry a unique energy and pride.

The downside of mixed practice is that the veterinarian is expected to know the latest information about all the diseases of all animal species. New information is constantly unfolding so this becomes an endless and frustrating task, particularly for solo practitioners who are already working seven days a week and available 24 hours a day. They are challenged with unusual diagnoses, difficult surgical procedures, and the need for specialized equipment.

General practitioners frequently refer patients to specialists for diagnostic procedures or surgery. These consultants may be privately practicing with their own offices or located at universities or state laboratories. It now appears that many general practitioners will be gradually replaced by species and discipline specialists both in private and public practice.

In addition to small animal practice, large animal practice, and mixed practice, there are numerous veterinary specialties which are practiced independently or in salaried positions in academe, government, or industry.

Gender Transition in Veterinary Medicine

Until the 1970s, veterinary medicine was a male-dominated profession. Most schools limited admission to one or possibly two women per class. The logic was based on the assumption that veterinarians mainly served farm animals and horses and that physical strength—in those days ascribed to masculinity—was essential for handling large animals. These assumptions proved untrue and the male exclusivity of veterinary medicine was challenged by the increase in small animal practices, by the women's rights movement, and by the demise of small family farms.

Women veterinarians always performed well in small animal practice and those who ventured into large animal medicine were as effective as men. As the word spread that women were being admitted to veterinary colleges and were being judged by the same standards as men, more and more women applied and were admitted.

The increasing number of women in the profession fits into the group practice concept in which multiple veterinarians join together in practice and everyone has some time off. This also provides part-time work that permits fulfillment of family responsibilities and time off for childbearing and rearing.

Women veterinarians mostly choose small animal practice, but some become equine specialists and some select mixed practice or species specialties in avian, bovine, ovine, caprine, or porcine medicine. An increasing number of women graduates have entered the profession over the years.

In this same period, America's population rapidly increased and the public became more aware of their relationships with their pets and more willing to invest in their health. Consequently, small animal practices blossomed and were visited more frequently. Women began assuming major roles in veterinary medicine.

This trend has gradually increased until now, approximately 80 percent of the nation's veterinary students are women and the percentage of women veterinarians is increasing each year.

The needs of women to have time off for caring for children accelerated the movement to group practices and the number of solo practitioners declined. While these changes were unfolding, the number of small animal practitioners and small animal specialties was rapidly expanding.

Diversity in Veterinary Medicine

After years of functioning as a white male profession, veterinary medicine has shifted to a female community. For many years, with a few exceptions, the profession made minimal efforts to attract diverse applicants to veterinary colleges.

In 2005, the Association of American Veterinary Medical Colleges (AAVMC) headquartered in Washington, DC, launched a major effort to recruit qualified under-represented minority students to its member colleges. This program encourages active recruitment programs, solicits scholarship funds, and develops data to bring the distribution of minority students, faculty, and graduates in the profession into alignment with the country's population with respect to race, color, and national origin.

AAVMC staff visit member colleges to encourage diversity measures. They also work with other health professions that share a similar challenge. Further information may be obtained at www.aavmc.org.

Veterinary Politics

Like most national and worldwide endeavors that blend the activities of people of varying interests, veterinary medicine cannot avoid involvement in personal and group affairs. These arise in the form of individual, internal, local, state, national, and global politics.

While there are always exceptions, the individual members of the veterinary profession are generally intelligent, dedicated, hard-working people who are respected by their friends, clients, and colleagues. Throughout their careers, they participate in a variety of veterinary organizations that work in various ways to strengthen the profession, upgrade its public image, and fund animal disease control programs and veterinary education.

Many veterinarians become involved in local politics and hold elected offices in organizations or governments and in other areas where it is impossible to please everyone. Others are active in state and national veterinary organizations that campaign to address issues in which veterinary perspectives are critical.

Relationships among veterinarians begin in veterinary college and sometimes earlier. The class sizes are usually small and most initial courses are attended by the entire class, so that like-thinking students often bond due to mutual commonalities. Most students soon know all their classmates by their first names. Occasionally students develop rivalries over class standing, class leadership positions, or personality differences.

A spirit of camaraderie is fostered early in their college days as veterinary students begin hearing that criticism of the professional judgment of colleagues is counterproductive, because everyone makes mistakes and the condition of patients will often change from day to day.

Often, companionships developed in veterinary college become lifelong friendships and sometimes result in partnerships in practice or other professional endeavors. Upon graduation some classmates stay in touch, but the newly graduated veterinarians mostly go their separate ways to face new sets of challenges and new political environments.

An initial challenge faced by new veterinarians is establishing positive relationships with neighboring veterinary colleagues. This is easy if a graduate joins a group practice. However, if a new veterinarian establishes a business in an area already occupied by established practitioners, a spirit of cooperation regarding fees, and a willingness to cooperate by alternating Sunday availability and vacation times, must be cooperatively worked out.

It takes particular effort to develop cooperative and noncompetitive relationships with neighboring veterinarians if they feel that their territory has been invaded. Once these details are resolved, neighboring practitioners can attend local veterinary meetings together and cooperate to serve the needs of the profession in their community.

Most veterinarians belong to state veterinary medical associations where they work together to serve the interests of the profession, promote ethical standards, and adjudicate occasional breaches of ethical codes.

At the state level, society leaders and members cultivate relationships with local and state legislators to expedite the quality of the profession, support laws that best serve animals and their owners, and that best address public health programs which relate to animals and animal-borne diseases of people.

Veterinarians who gain leadership positions at the state level often take a step upward and become actively involved in species or discipline specialty organizations at the national level. These organizations provide educational opportunities, present updates on developments in their fields, and express concerns to nationally influential organizations and legislative bodies.

In addition to state veterinary medical societies, there are influential national veterinary organizations like the AVMA, the United States Animal Health Association (USAHA), and the AAVMC that actively lobby federal legislators on matters about which veterinarians are knowledgeable. These include public health issues, international trade regulations, funding for animal health research, and veterinary education.

The global interests of veterinary medicine are represented by many organizations and many government veterinary leaders. These individuals represent the interests of the country at various international trade coalitions and meetings of the World Organisation for Animal Health (OIE).

Veterinary Vaccines and Drugs

An amazing number of animal vaccines and drugs are available to veterinarians, and some of these are sold to the general public. The prevailing rule about vaccinations is that no vaccine is 100 percent effective and no vaccine is 100 percent safe. Vaccines licensed in the US are as safe and effective as current technology permits. Vaccine technology is continually advancing.

The safety, effectiveness (efficacy), and labeling of US veterinary vaccines is overseen by the US Department of Agriculture (USDA). The USDA's Center for Veterinary Biologics, which is located at the National Veterinary Services Laboratory in Ames, Iowa, conducts product testing. The USDA also inspects animal vaccine production facilities.

The AVMA has an elected Council on Biologic and Therapeutic Agents which supplies practitioner, academic, and corporate input into the regulation of veterinary vaccines. Veterinary practitioners are responsible for seeing that vaccines are properly handled, stored, and administered according to label requirements to assure maximum safety and effectiveness.

The safety and efficacy of animal drugs other than vaccines is overseen, supervised, and regulated by the US Food and Drug Administration (FDA), which is an agency of the US Department of Health and Human Services. The FDA Center for Veterinary Medicine approves drugs used on each animal species and regulates the dosages, routes of administration, the indications for their use, and the withdrawal times required before treated animals and their products (such as eggs and milk) can be used as food.

A Complex and Well-Respected Profession

The characteristics described above make veterinary medicine a unique and well-respected profession that is admired throughout the world. This positive public image of veterinarians has contributed to the expanding numbers of applicants to colleges of veterinary medicine and to the continual advancement of the profession.

CHAPTER 2
COLLEGES OF VETERINARY MEDICINE

Introduction

There are 28 accredited US colleges of veterinary medicine (CVMs) located in 26 states, and four Canadian CVMs. They share many commonalities. In addition to awarding the Doctor of Veterinary Medicine degree, the US and Canadian veterinary colleges have similar curriculums and schedules.

US Colleges of Veterinary Medicine

The 28 US CVMs and schools of veterinary medicine (SVMs) provide opportunities for residents of 28 states. California and Alabama each house two veterinary colleges and Maryland and Virginia share a regional college at Virginia Tech University. This leaves 22 states without a CVM. Some of these states arrange contracts with nearby states to admit a quota of their students in exchange for payments to offset the costs.

Aspiring students who reside in states without a CVM must apply to universities in other states, and most US colleges accept some nonresident students. States without a veterinary college are frequently urged to provide one, but after investigating the costs and challenges involved they decide to proceed without one.

US colleges of veterinary medicine are carefully monitored by the Council on Education (COE) of the American Veterinary Medical Association (AVMA), which accredits each US CVM based on acceptable facilities, faculties, and curriculums. The COE conducts periodic site visits and reviews detailed self-study reports prepared by each college.

Most states require a degree from an accredited college of veterinary medicine to qualify for a license to practice within their boundaries. Licenses are usually awarded after applicants pass required state or national board examinations.

There are nonaccredited veterinary colleges in the Caribbean, the West Indies, and elsewhere whose graduates can qualify to practice in some states after passing a designated examination for foreign veterinary graduates. When foreign veterinary graduates pass this examination, most states still require that they pass national or their own state board examinations for licensure. Many graduates of foreign veterinary schools maintain highly qualified practices in the US.

The 28 US veterinary colleges are:

- Auburn University CVM, Auburn, AL;
- Tuskegee University School of Veterinary Medicine (SVM), Tuskegee, AL;
- University of California SVM, Davis, CA;
- Western University School of Health Sciences CVM, Pomona, CA;
- Colorado State University CVM & Biomedical Sciences, Fort Collins, CO;
- University of Florida CVM, Gainesville, FL;
- University of Georgia CVM, Athens, GA;
- University of Illinois CVM, Urbana, IL;
- Purdue University SVM, West Lafayette, IN;
- Iowa State University CVM, Ames, IA;
- Kansas State University CVM, Manhattan, KS;
- Louisiana State University SVM, Baton Rouge, LA;
- Cummings School of Veterinary Medicine, Tufts University, East Grafton, MA;
- Michigan State University CVM, East Lansing, MI;
- University of Minnesota CVM, Saint Paul, MN;
- Mississippi State University CVM, Mississippi State, MS;
- University of Missouri CVM, Columbia, MO;
- Cornell University CVM, Ithaca, NY;
- North Carolina State University CVM, Raleigh, NC;
- The Ohio State University CVM, Columbus, OH;
- Oklahoma State University Center for Veterinary Health Sciences, Stillwater, OK;
- Oregon State University CVM, Corvallis, OR;
- University of Pennsylvania SVM, Philadelphia, PA;
- University of Tennessee CVM, Knoxville, TN;
- Texas A&M University CVM and Biomedical Sciences, College Station, TX;
- Virginia Tech and University of Maryland, Virginia-Maryland Regional CVM, Blacksburg, VA;

- Washington State University CVM, Pullman, WA; and
- University of Wisconsin-Madison School of VM, Madison, WS.

Canadian Colleges of Veterinary Medicine

The Canadian colleges of veterinary medicine are:

- The University of Montreal Faculty of Veterinary Medicine in Saint-Hyacinthe, Quebec;
- The Ontario Veterinary College in Guelph, Ontario;
- The University of Prince Edward Island Atlantic Veterinary College in Charlottetown, Prince Edward Island; and
- The University of Saskatchewan, Western College of Veterinary Medicine in Saskatoon, Saskatchewan.

Occasionally, citizens cross national borders to attend or work at a CVM or participate in corporate activities. The Canadian vet colleges work closely with US veterinary schools and have relatively similar admission requirements, curriculums, and faculties.

Variable Admission Requirements

Each CVM or SVM has its own admission requirements and these requirements vary between colleges. Most have nonrefundable application fees. They also have differing curriculums, facilities, tuition and fees, and areas of academic emphasis. These variables all change gradually over the years, so current information is essential for applicants. This can usually be obtained by visiting a college's website.

Most colleges of veterinary medicine require a minimum of two years of college-level, pre-veterinary studies. These prerequisites comprise a variety of courses such as animal science, biology, biochemistry, chemistry, computer science, physics, social and physical sciences, mathematics, and zoology. These pre-veterinary requirements usually must be accompanied by a broad background in general education including English.

Most successful applicants have completed the requirements for a bachelor's degree and many have had some graduate level courses before entering veterinary college. It is important to have completed the required college courses for an institution before submitting an application. Information about required courses can usually be obtained from the individual colleges or from the Veterinary Medical College Application Service (VMCAS) via the Internet at www.aavmc.org.

Veterinary College Curriculums

The curriculums of colleges of veterinary medicine are determined by faculty curriculum committees. Most curriculums are flexible but they must meet accreditation requirements established by the Council on Education (COE) of the American Veterinary Medical Association (AVMA). Most schools have a basic core of required courses that conform to AVMA guidelines. They usually have electives that correspond to faculty preferences, student interests, and the nature of local livestock and pet populations.

Most Doctor of Veterinary Medicine (DVM) degree programs comprise three years of classroom instruction and a year of clinical rotations in the fourth (senior) year. However, some schools introduce a taste of hands-on clinical instruction throughout the first three years, and there are many modifications of that model. Class content changes constantly as new information emerges, as new courses are added, and as faculty members change.

Even longstanding courses that are taught by a single professor will change as the instructor develops unique interests and approaches. Many courses are taught by multiple faculty members who each teach one portion of the course and who usually don't hear their colleagues' presentations. Thus there can be repetition, and, occasionally, conflicting ideas are presented. However, multiple-professor courses add a variety of emphases to the curriculum.

Veterinary College Facilities

The buildings and facilities of veterinary colleges vary considerably. However, they must conform to the requirements of both the home university and the COE.

Veterinary college facilities usually involve offices, classrooms, laboratories, and hospitals that support administrative, teaching, clinical, diagnostic, and research activities. Most veterinary colleges also house extension personnel who disseminate updated animal health information to livestock owners, pet owners, and veterinarians.

The need for hospitals with facilities for diagnostic, medical, and surgical procedures which can accommodate pet animals as well as all avian, bovine, caprine, equine, ovine, and porcine species, makes veterinary educational facilities expensive. These costs are amplified by the need for isolation facilities for animals with infectious diseases, some of which are transmissible to people.

Veterinary College Faculties

Most veterinary faculties are diverse mixtures of experts in various areas of the college's teaching, research, and extension missions.

Usually, all faculty members in the clinical sciences (those that address animal patients) are veterinarians. Faculty members in research and basic sciences, such as biochemistry, immunology, microbiology, and physiology, may have PhD degrees but are not necessarily veterinarians. The AVMA accreditation requirements state that the dean of each college of veterinary medicine must be a veterinarian. Most courses that deal with the diagnosis, treatment, and prevention of animal diseases, or with clinical medicine or surgery are taught by veterinarians.

Faculties are usually more diverse with respect to race, gender, and national origins than the student bodies, which are largely comprised of white females. An occasional challenge arises when students cannot understand lectures given by foreign faculty members with heavy accents.

Selecting Veterinary Colleges

It is sometimes difficult to determine the areas of academic, clinical, and research emphasis at each veterinary college because differing individuals will present varying opinions about a college's priorities. Most colleges profess that they devote equal emphasis to basic academic enterprises, patient care, extension programs, professional preparation, and research. Persons in the know often differ with such proclamations.

In some colleges there is a feeling that teaching excellence, particularly in clinical fields, is rewarded less than success in research and grant acquisition. These rewards involve the hiring process, salaries, promotions, and the granting of faculty tenure.

With particular interests in mind when selecting the veterinary colleges to which to submit applications, one can find it difficult to determine differences from the websites and college brochures. Information is best obtained from folks with inside knowledge. Costs are an important factor.

Usually, if your home state has a veterinary college, it pays to apply there and to several others. The most highly populated states usually receive the most applications and thus have smaller percentages of successful applicants.

All the US and Canadian colleges that are listed above are accredited by the AVMA. Applications are best submitted to these colleges because most states require degrees from AVMA accredited colleges as a prerequisite for taking their licensing examinations. Graduates of nonaccredited veterinary colleges must undergo additional exams and graduates of some foreign schools must go through clinical rotations in an accredited college before beginning the US licensing process.

Accredited Colleges of Veterinary Medicine

As indicated above, all US and Canadian colleges of veterinary medicine are currently accredited by the AVMA COE. Some foreign accredited colleges include the Universities of Edinburgh and Glasgow in Scotland, the University of London, Massey University in New Zealand, Murdock University and the University of Melbourne in Australia, and the University of Utrecht in the Netherlands.

Members of the AVMA Council on Education are elected by the AVMA House of Delegates. The council has the authority to evaluate colleges and assign them an accreditation classification.

The accreditation process is complex and there are several levels of accreditation. These accreditation classifications are based on the council's evaluation of each college's organization and mission statement and on assurance that it has status and autonomy similar to other colleges in the home university system.

Colleges must possess adequate administrative staff, finances, and physical facilities including teaching hospitals, teaching and research laboratories, classrooms, and offices. They must have adequate normal, healthy animals, hospital patients, and library facilities for teaching purposes. They must also provide public information about their admission policies. The admission policies must be spelled out and be administered by a committee containing mostly full-time faculty members.

The four-year veterinary curriculum should include at least one academic year of hands-on clinical experience. The clinical courses should include multiple animal species and a variety of diseases and diagnostic challenges. By graduation, students must have familiarity with the role of veterinarians in animal and human health, food safety, and zoonotic diseases. Research activities must be integrated with the professional programs.

Based on the above factors, examination of each college's annual reports, and the results of site visits, the COE assigns an accreditation status to each college. The possible accreditations include: Reasonable Assurance, Provisional Accreditation, Full Accreditation, Limited Accreditation, or Terminal Accreditation.

Challenges Facing Veterinary Colleges

Veterinary colleges in the US and Canada all face significant challenges in upcoming years. These challenges include the increasingly high cost per student, rapidly emerging new information, fixed perceptions of the profession by entering students, ever increasing numbers of qualified applicants, and the changing interests of graduates.

High Costs per Student

The high costs per student of veterinary education are imposed upon both the universities with veterinary colleges and upon the students themselves.

The **university expenses** for colleges of veterinary medicine are among the highest of academic disciplines because of the need to provide unique clinical and hospital facilities so that each student can gain hands-on clinical experience with all species of animals.

The possibility of reducing these costs is challenged by entrenched academic policies, the requirements for maintaining accreditation, and firm beliefs that every veterinarian must have knowledge and college-supplied background in all diseases, injuries, and surgical procedures for all animal species. Some colleges are addressing these challenges with flexible curriculums, elective opportunities, and by exchanging faculty and students for the study of diseases of various animal species, a process sometimes called "tracking."

Student-incurred expenses at colleges of veterinary medicine are similar to other college programs but are imposed during years when most other students have already completed their college education. Thus, veterinary students frequently incur multiple debts from the costs of extra years of travel, tuition, fees, rooms, and meals. Throughout all phases of college education, these expenses are causing a revolution in thinking about college among families at all income levels.

The costs of attending different colleges of veterinary medicine vary considerably. In general, particularly at state universities, tuition is less expensive for residents than for out-of-state individuals, unless there is a contract between the home state of the applicant and the out-of-state university.

College expenses can be ameliorated by loans and scholarships offered by the colleges, outside organizations, and individuals. Loans are easy to obtain, but grants and scholarships require diligent searching. Costs can also be moderated by thrifty habits, dressing conservatively, eating inexpensively, and buying second-hand books. Some veterinary students seek outside jobs or work for room or board, but these activities are best delayed until the individuals have adjusted to their curriculums and schedules.

Rapidly Emerging New information

There are increasing volumes of new animal health information, much of which is pertinent to the activities of the veterinary profession, and a small portion of which sometimes seems irrelevant but involves information which faculty feel should be included in the curriculum.

Some of this new information may dilute the importance of hands-on experience and real-world experience needed for public service, assistance to pet animals and livestock, and dealing with zoonotic diseases and food safety issues.

Some people feel that theoretical information imposes extra years of college training on people who largely perform relatively routine activities requiring talents which could be acquired in less time. This perplexing dilemma is countered by the fact that however routine, certain levels of understanding are essential to properly understand the realities and contraindications of procedures as simple as vaccinations, and the observations and examinations that should precede them.

Fixed Perceptions of Entering Students

Despite the profession's efforts to acquaint students with the many essential societal roles played by veterinarians, the general public and applicants to colleges of veterinary medicine remain relatively naïve about the versatility of the profession.

People are surprised that veterinarians address public health, food safety, prevention of zoonotic diseases, development and evaluation of pharmaceutical and biological products, the control of international movement of livestock and livestock products, and procurement of foodstuffs for US troops in other nations.

The profession has been collectively introverted with respect to publicizing their participation in these essential programs and enthusiastically introducing them into professional curriculums.

Increasing Numbers of Applicant Rejections

As the US population increases, the number of applicants to veterinary colleges is rising and more aspiring veterinarians must be rejected. Some rejected applicants become disenchanted and might actively criticize the profession, its admission policies, and its academic procedures.

Some possible alleviating measures could include increasing class sizes, opening new colleges of veterinary medicine, adjusting curricular and licensing procedures to permit species-limited graduates to graduate and be licensed, and developing computer-based courses and licensing examinations for those wishing to add additional species to their practice qualifications.

The Changing Interests of Graduates

There is a pattern of changing focus of veterinary students and graduates with respect to practice type, species preferences, and specialty selection.

Today most veterinary students begin their veterinary education with small animal practice as a goal. However, a program that teaches small animal medicine exclusively would create deficiencies for the 40 percent of veterinarians who decide within 20 years after graduation that they wish to pursue another aspect of the profession.

The Dynamics of Veterinary Education

Colleges of veterinary medicine in the US and around the world are aware of the issues addressed above and are moving toward a variety of solutions.

Many proposed remedies involve money and will require support of state and federal legislatures. Despite these challenges, veterinary medicine remains one of the most trusted, respected, and desired professions.

Students who are interested in veterinary medicine and wish to pursue careers requiring professional integrity and professional credibility are encouraged to pursue this ambition with enthusiasm and vigor.

CHAPTER 3
LONG-TERM STRATEGIES FOR POTENTIAL APPLICANTS

Introduction

The idea of being a veterinarian can arise in many ways, including loving a pet, riding horses, or by observing animals in parades, at zoos, or on farms.

Young people considering careers in veterinary medicine are contemplating a future that requires thought, dedication, and energy. When youth undertake activities they hope will lead to admission to a veterinary college, they embark on a path that qualifies them for many other fields.

Successful admission to a veterinary college requires a singular mindset that should be established as early as possible. This attitude converts individuals who might not normally emphasize education in their teens, to serious students with strong personal ideals.

This mindset requires committed effort on the part of young people considering applying to colleges of veterinary medicine. Their efforts also need support and encouragement from their parents, teachers, coaches, and mentors of all sorts. This chapter begins with suggestions for potential applicants and includes comments on the role of adults in encouraging their efforts.

Once young people decide they want to be veterinarians, it is time for them to begin plotting a course of action to increase their odds of admission to a veterinary college.

If started early enough, the following plan will launch a new lifestyle that will raise their grades, improve their academic standing, elevate their standard test scores, assure acceptance into a variety of colleges, and make them competitive applicants for colleges of veterinary medicine.

A Basis for Successful Applications

Veterinary medicine is a career that is often identified at an early age. When this occurs, it is appropriate to encourage youthful ambitions and help young people to increase their chances of successful admission to a college of veterinary medicine. Successful applications are easiest for those with a passion for the profession, who have announced their ambition early. The following advice provides a basis for success in veterinary medicine and many other careers.

Develop Traits Favoring Admission

During the preteen and teenage years, there are many opportunities to plot a course toward successful admission to a veterinary college. While it is tempting to hang out and have fun, your veterinary ambitions will be best served by a shift toward scholarship, productive activities, character building, and personal development. Don't pass up these opportunities; they are all part of becoming a veterinarian and undertaking careers in a variety of other fields.

Applicants who select the profession while in college can get admitted to veterinary colleges. However, the more effort spent on developing an acceptable admission background, the better the chances are. Begin to develop some animal savvy and a scholarship package based on the following activities:

- observing veterinarians and animals;
- spending a summer on a farm;
- reading books about veterinary medicine;
- talking about your veterinary goals;
- developing a passion for education;
- working hard at school;
- participating in extracurricular activities;
- accepting nominations for class offices;
- striving for high standard test scores; and
- working on reading, writing, and speaking.

If you are a prospective veterinarian, the activities and efforts detailed below will increase your appreciation of the profession, sharpen your intellect, and position you for future academic successes.

Observe Veterinarians at Work

Seeing a veterinarian successfully save an ailing animal or skillfully perform a surgical procedure could ignite a career obsession. Ask local veterinarians if you may observe them at work. If granted that opportunity, watch carefully, be quiet, stay out of the way, and volunteer to help with tasks like picking up, sweeping floors, cleaning kennels, and running errands.

Observe veterinarians carefully and keep in mind that one individual's efforts are only a tiny part of the many services that the profession performs. If you decide that what they do is not for you, locate another veterinarian and try again.

Read Books about Veterinary Medicine

There are lots of books about veterinarians and veterinary medicine.[1] Read some books that provide insights into the many aspects of the profession and see if you really want to pursue it. Books about different kinds of animals, their habits, their diets, and their relationship with people also will inspire you. Although slightly technical, *The Merck Veterinary Manual*[2] is informative and complete in its coverage of the profession.

Spend a Summer on a Farm

Part of veterinary medicine involves farm animals. Whether or not you decide you want to work with livestock, working on a farm and getting some experience with livestock will expand your understanding of the profession—and add a few points to your application.

If you live on a farm your home experience will help, but it might broaden your perspective to do some work for neighboring farmers. If you reside in a rural area it should be easy to find a low-paying but useful farm job. If you dwell in an urban or suburban area, try to find someone who can put you in touch with a farmer who needs summer help. You will be glad you did.

Talk about Your Veterinary Goals

Without dominating conversations or interrupting, tell your friends, relatives, teachers, and other people about your wish to be a veterinarian. They will inevitably tell you of their experience with veterinarians and you will find out many things you were previously unaware of. Let them talk while you listen carefully. They may know veterinarians who will let you observe them at work and who will tell you things about the profession that will assist you in deciding if that is what you really want.

Don't be surprised if some people tell you that you'll never make it. When hearing that, just say quietly to yourself, "I will show them," and vow to work even harder.

Develop a Passion for Education

Remember that your application for admission will be evaluated by educators (veterinary college faculty). Generally, people excel at things for which they have a sincere passion. In public schools, kids with a passion for education are rare because peer pressure drives them in other directions.

It takes extreme effort, particularly by those for whom education has been a struggle, to decide to switch gears, start studying, and to move upward in class standings.

Work Hard at School

Veterinary medicine is only one of many fulfilling careers that require extra educational efforts. It is essential to become studious as early as possible. In the United States, the road to college is via high school, a route which is available free of charge to everyone.

There are probably many classmates now making better grades than you, and with little or no effort. The secret is to shift into high gear as early as possible, ideally in elementary school, next best in middle school or junior high school, and definitely by high school. This demands an ambitious attack on the challenges of schoolwork, studying every day, and learning as much as possible about reading, writing, spelling, math, and science.

High gear requires that instead of hanging out and watching TV, you conquer the books, listen carefully in class, study every night, and use your untapped innate potential to prepare for that dream lifetime that you might think is out of your reach. This does not mean you must become a hermit. You can also enjoy extracurricular activities and learn to carefully choose spare-time activities that are relaxing and trouble-free.

Good grades in school are one measure of accomplishment and are preparation for a satisfying, productive, and prosperous future. While some students have genetic or parentally ingrained characteristics that expedite learning, most people and many students are unaware that the US school systems are set up to accommodate all students. Thus, youngsters from all backgrounds can succeed if they work at it.

This success requires effort, and some youngsters must work harder than others. There are advantages and disadvantages to being among those who need to struggle to achieve. Those who struggle develop the ability to concentrate, to focus on concepts as well as details, to succeed in other activities like writing, playing musical instruments, or sports, where practice and repetition are major keys to success.

The disadvantage of having to work hard is that unless a passion is present, it is very easy to accept the idea that one is not intelligent or gifted enough to meet the challenges. That belief doesn't acknowledge the fact that the average person uses only about 15 percent of their innate ability. Students and their mentors must realize their tremendous potential and should not let inner voices or external pressures convince them otherwise.

Participate in Extracurricular Activities

A balanced mix of academic excellence and success in extracurricular activities such as band, chorus, cheerleading, debate, drama, scouting, sports, yearbook, or other programs suggests a well-rounded individual with potential to adapt to multiple situations. College admission committees are known to seek academically acceptable candidates with a variety of experiences.

Here is a note to parents: A few words of congratulations for increased study can provide a kickoff for continued successes. When kids are told that they are great, it boosts their morale and inspires further achievement of the kind needed to succeed as a veterinarian.

Young people considering veterinary careers should participate enthusiastically in activities that utilize the magnificent energy that many teenagers can waste on nonproductive endeavors.

Accept Nominations for Class Offices

If you work to develop outstanding interpersonal skills, you will eventually be asked if someone may nominate you for some position. Without being pushy or grossly political, gladly accept any nomination to run for an office at school, church, or in any organization in which you participate.

If elected, thank those who may have voted for you and work diligently to perform the duties of the position. However small it seems, it will provide valuable experience and will look good on your college applications.

Strive for High Standard Test Scores

Standard test scores are one part of admissions criteria for most colleges. These tests are administered in high school and in college. They include the Scholastic Aptitude Test (SAT), the American College Test (ACT), and the Graduate Record Exam (GRE). Information about these tests can be accessed on the Internet where examples of test questions and study guides are available.

The SAT and ACT are usually taken in high school for use with college entrance applications. The GRE is usually taken in college to indicate ability to succeed in graduate programs. The GRE is a requirement for application to many veterinary colleges.

Junior high school is not too early to begin thinking about these tests and trying some questions to detect areas where increased efforts are needed. This preparation will strengthen your opportunity for higher education in all areas. Ask your teachers to give you some old standard test questions. Look them over and decide to work daily to increase your capacity to do well on them.

Work on Reading, Writing, and Speaking

Three attributes shared by most successful individuals are reading, writing, and speaking. Strangely, these are all skills which young people shun in the years when they are most easily cultivated. To avoid embarrassment, they hide the fact that they feel insufficient in one or more of these skills. However, if they tell a teacher that they think they need help in some area, it will usually be provided.

Successful college-level work requires rapid reading with high levels of comprehension. Secrets to reading improvement are available in library books and on the Internet.

Similarly, writing is readily improved by studying some of the many books on writing that are available in libraries, on the Internet, and on the bargain shelves in bookstores. Teachers can also help with writing. Writing differs markedly from speaking.[3, 4]

Everyday speaking expands your vocabulary and provides opportunities to practice good English. Your parents have your best interest at heart when they correct your pronunciation and your use of language. Good English is essential for professional success and for clear writing.

Public speaking puts fear into the minds of many people but is an easily developed skill that can be cultivated by taking the Dale Carnegie Course or by joining in the supportive environment of a local Toastmasters club. Toastmasters clubs can be easily located at www.toastmasters.org. Speaking skills which are cultivated early will be noticed by others and will stimulate new levels of confidence.

The addition of reading, writing, and speaking excellence to your current abilities will strengthen your personality, confidence, enthusiasm, and interpersonal skills and will impress individuals who will be writing letters of recommendation for you.

The Importance of Interpersonal Skills

While working to increase your academic prowess, you will probably find some new friends and seek opportunities to shape a new personality which is consistent with the traits required for admission to veterinary college and practice of the profession. These requirements demand that you:

- perfect your interpersonal skills;
- develop a personal code of ethics;
- sidestep trouble;
- develop integrity and credibility;
- pay attention to your health;
- tap your unlimited potential;
- politely decline tobacco, alcohol, and drugs;
- limit TV time and selections; and
- consider alternative career choices.

Efforts directed to develop a professionally positive, ethical, and respected personality using the following suggestions will pay off throughout your lifetime.

Develop Interpersonal Skills

Positive interactions with people of all ages help develop sound relationships and the respect of everyone who knows you. Positive attitudes, smiles, and sincere efforts to have people share their accomplishments and concerns with you are fundamental to establishing friendships and for consideration of leadership positions.

When you are sincerely interested in the progress that others are making and correspondingly less occupied with promoting your own accomplishments, people will recognize you as a friend and colleague, remember you, and recommend you for awards and other recognition. When you listen carefully to the thoughts and concerns of others—instead of interrupting to interject your own experiences—you may be the only person who exhibited any interest or concern about their activities in several days and you will have a new friend.

Pleasant interpersonal skills can be developed by following the advice put forward in the books of Dale Carnegie.[5]

Develop a Personal Code of Ethics

Ethical behavior is essential for professional success. It requires a sense of right and wrong and a dedication to credibility and integrity. The American Veterinary Medical Association (AVMA) has a set of published *Principles of Veterinary Medical Ethics.*

This code (see page 141) is published in the *AVMA Membership Directory & Resource Manual*[7] which can be perused in the offices of local veterinarians. It provides guidelines for professional conduct. The AVMA encourages all state and local veterinary associations to use these principles for developing local codes of ethics.

The basic elements of the code are honesty, fairness, considerateness, compassion, responsibility, and application of a professional attitude, behavior, and appearance. While they are spelled out in terms specific to professional activities, they include models of conduct that are appropriate for all interactions with people and animals.

Potential applicants would benefit from studying the AVMA ethics code and adopting it as a personal guideline while still in elementary, middle, or high school. The principles in this code will serve you well regardless of your ultimate career. The golden rule, DO UNTO OTHERS AS YOU WOULD HAVE THEM DO UNTO YOU, is the basis for this code and for most successful human interactions.

A reputation for personal ethics following this model will be of value to anyone applying for admission to a college of veterinary medicine. Applicants must sincerely cherish and work to develop and protect a reputation for honesty, integrity, and for appreciation for and consideration of the rights of others.

Sidestep Trouble

Young people rarely realize that the problems created in early years by persuasive "fun-seeking" companions can create a reputation as a troublemaker, delinquent, or loudmouth, and can surface later as negative verbal and written evaluations. Young people considering veterinary careers don't need such reputations.

Trouble is best avoided by listening carefully to the plans of youthful companions. When a suggested escapade has the slightest hint of trouble, simply insist that you need to be home, and depart the scene.

Develop Integrity and Credibility

Integrity is unquestioned sincerity, honesty, and belief that every thought, word, and deed exemplifies an individual's character. Credibility is defined as trustworthiness. While they are very similar in their meanings, these two words (credibility and integrity) traditionally partner to summarize the characteristics essential to professionals and others whom the public can rely on.

If prospective veterinarians wish to have teachers, mentors, and neighbors recommend them for a profession in which personal integrity and professional credibility are keystones, they must bear these qualities in mind whenever they think, speak, or act.

Tap Your Unlimited Potential

There are numerous criteria for applying to and entering the pathways of professions and occupations. These require that students, once they select a career, must be encouraged to awaken to the vastness of their potential. Their possibilities for success are largely unsuspected by young people because mediocrity has been ingrained in their minds as an inevitable fact.

Hopefully, potential veterinarians will be alerted that if support and encouragement are not forthcoming from parents, teachers, and other mentors, they can still succeed by taking matters into their own hands and embarking on a path to show everyone what they can do. This involves considerable effort yet is worthwhile.

Exploitation of one's unlimited potential can be accomplished unilaterally if support is not forthcoming. Progress toward capturing hidden talents may not be initially recognized or praised by others and may even result in teasing from classmates. However, in the long run, this personal progress will leave you in the driver's seat to choose a rewarding career while your critics are less happy and successful. Unleashing your potential may lead to election as a team captain or class officer. These strategies can be applied at all levels of life.

Pay Attention to Your Health

Few young people realize that improved success inevitably arises in all activities undertaken by a healthy body which receives adequate sleep, exercise, and nutrition. Extra rest is needed during adolescent growth years. Hard work in school, if followed by some exciting extracurricular activities, is enough to overcome insomnia by early evening.

Investing time and effort to achieve academic and extracurricular excellence requires a well-rested and invigorated body and mind. This is accomplished with adequate sleep, an appropriate diet, and physical fitness. It is essential to avoid obesity resulting from excess consumption of fats, sweets, and snacks. Eat three well-balanced meals daily and avoid eating between meals, take a multivitamin-mineral pill daily, and exercise regularly.

Along with this routine, determine the time of day when you function most effectively and when you feel most rested. If you are a morning person, begin rising early and study while others sleep. If you function more effectively at night, seek a nighttime hideaway for study.

Explore your body style to see how much sleep you need for maximum efficiency. Determine if a nap after lunch helps or hinders your effectiveness. Keep an eye on weekend activities to assure that they don't interrupt an otherwise efficiently functioning system. Eat and drink in moderation and take nothing in excess. This motto is best followed by totally avoiding alcohol, tobacco, and drugs.

Politely Decline Alcohol, Tobacco, and Drugs

Alcohol, tobacco, and drugs are addicting substances that can take over your life and cripple you physically, mentally, and financially. Users of addictive substances constantly urge others to join them, possibly because they are aware that they are decimating their minds and bodies and don't want to be alone in the undertaking.

The only thing the first taste of these substances can accomplish is to make you hunger for more. As you mature you will recognize hundreds of friends and relatives whose health, wealth, relationships, and wisdom have been permanently sabotaged by addictions. When invited to partake, decline politely with a nonjudgmental but firm "No, thanks."

Limit TV Time and Selections

When wondering where you will get the time to prepare yourself for applying to veterinary college, take a hard look at the time spent in front of the television set, playing computer games, and hanging out.

Some carefully chosen TV programs provide a global awareness and a broad background of knowledge—including information about animals. However, many TV activities are a waste of time that impose a sense of negativity, and some can affect your attentiveness and ability to concentrate.

You can add precious minutes to your daily study time by carefully selecting truly valuable TV programs and recording them so they can be watched at a chosen time and fast-forwarded through the commercials.

It is only years later when many people realize that the TV time could been have better spent and that the colleagues who spent time studying or participating in productive activities ended up happier, more prosperous, and more secure.

Television has some wonderful and appropriate programs, but it is a chore to find and watch them when one is also confronted with the violent and dramatic, but dangerously addictive, programming and commercials that stimulate negativity and nonproductive, habit-forming lifestyles.

Consider Alternative Career Choices

While seriously considering veterinary medicine, look at other career choices. There are many—including medicine, nursing, pharmacy, veterinary technology, teaching, and law—that require similar preparation. The previously described goals can help with many worthwhile and rewarding career options which can let you bypass the alternative (chosen by many schoolmates) to wind up working at dead-end jobs.

Career Strategies at Various Stages of Life

Developmental strategies for admission to veterinary college and other career choices sometimes emerge automatically for a few very talented and lucky individuals. For most people aspiring to become veterinarians, these strategies must be recognized and consciously cultivated throughout early life and into college. This requires individual effort and parental and mentor support in cultivating productive habits and skills as early as possible. The following sections describe the essential roles of parents and other mentors.

Parental and Other Adult Guidance

The support of parents, relatives, teachers, coaches, scoutmasters, and other advisors and mentors is a vital portion of preparation for the challenging task of gaining admission to schools and colleges of veterinary medicine. Once a young person verbally expresses interest in becoming a veterinarian, the need for support and encouragement is essential.

If parents, teachers, and coaches query them about what they want to do as adults, encouraging comments can lead young people to seek a pathway to a variety of goals. You may have heard rumors that admission to veterinary colleges is virtually impossible because they have ten times more applicants than they have room for and that successful admission requires academic genius, excellent recommendations, a charming personality, political connections, financial backing, and a lot of luck.

Some of these suppositions come from people who applied unsuccessfully to a veterinary college and were embittered by the process. Some unsuccessful veterinary college applicants resent the profession and carry a dislike for veterinarians. The general public rarely hears their comments until someone expresses interest in going to veterinary college and is then bombarded with negative and discouraging remarks from a rejected applicant.

Such commentary can be countered by the proposition that veterinary medicine is a highly respected profession. In fact, when people are told someone is a veterinarian, they sometimes say "You are a veterinarian? Wow!" or utter similar expressions of admiration and awe.

Encouragement in Grade School

Grade school might seem early to start preparing to apply to veterinary colleges. However, once the student makes that decision, parents and other mentors can start encouraging them.

Their mentors can help by impressing on them that educational quality is one major determinant of their future destiny in this age of technology.

The attention and effort developed in elementary school sets the stage for future achievements. By the time they reach 10 to 12 years old, many youngsters are talking about being veterinarians and they deserve support and encouragement whether they end up as veterinarians or as something quite different.

Therefore, positive, non-nagging incentives to listen and learn, to expand their vocabularies and learning skills, and to tap into their innate potential are essential. Positive reinforcement sets a course for success in grade school, middle or junior high school, high school, and in all future endeavors including veterinary medicine.

Because Americans utilize only about 15 percent of their intellectual and creative capacity, all children are capable of rising to upper levels in their classes if positively motivated, stimulated, and rewarded for their efforts.

One often neglected learning component is writing. Many children despise and postpone writing. This is unfortunate because for many people writing is the peak of a learning pyramid comprised of hearing, seeing, reading, experiencing, talking, and writing about a subject.[3, 4]

If young people can develop good writing skills without being hounded or badgered by parents and teachers, they have an advantage in the learning process. This is a delicate matter; negative comments about a student's writing ability are usually counterproductive.

Telling grade school students to begin preparing for admission to veterinary college sounds unrealistic. However, the reality is that once students express interest, parental guidance, teacher inspiration, and hard work at any level can lay the groundwork for a variety of successful careers and ultimately determine the basis of future academic successes that can lead to careers with satisfying and rewarding occupations.

Admittedly, it is extremely difficult to set elementary school students on a course of academic success if they are unable or unwilling to proceed. Nonetheless, asking them what they want to do when they grow up, and positively pointing out the value of successful learning at an early age, are helpful steps.

Awakenings during middle school and high school are not always too late to set a course leading to admission to veterinary colleges or other careers requiring college-level training. There is often a remarkable change in class standings between elementary school and high school based on changing maturity, incentives, positive reinforcement, and each young person's decisions regarding the future.

Middle School and Junior High School

Middle school and junior high school are times when kids unconsciously set the stage for lifetime achievements. During this period, behavioral styles, attention levels, and study and learning patterns are becoming established and are usually still easily modified.

Without nagging, teachers and mentors can positively reinforce kids' comments about future professions with an absence of "can't and don't"; an abundance of "can dos"; and with realistic suggestions about seeking opinion-molding experiences both in school and elsewhere. At these ages, students' contacts with animals, veterinarians, farmers, and kennel owners are valuable.

Middle school and junior high school students need support and encouragement to upgrade their learning styles with concentration on things that appear irrelevant at that age. This requires repetition of definitions and practice in spelling, reading, and writing.

Parents without college educations need to work particularly hard to convince their kids of the opportunities that they themselves missed and how their offspring can capitalize on current opportunities in which their parents didn't participate.

High School

High school—which sets the stage for college admission—is an excellent setting for establishing essential backgrounds for future success and happiness. During high school days, few youngsters give thought to career opportunities.

An awakening in high school is almost essential because of its impact on admission to a relatively rigorous college at which to undertake pre-veterinary studies.

While still in high school, aspiring veterinary students must select colleges where they will pursue pre-veterinary studies and be sure they offer the courses required by their chosen veterinary colleges.

College

College experience is important because colleges of veterinary medicine have strict collegiate pre-veterinary requirements. If the veterinary profession is still a goal after high school, the selection of required college-level, pre-veterinary courses is critical.

When comparing college grades, most veterinary college admission committees consider the academic standing of the programs in which the scores were achieved. They also examine other predictors of success in a strenuous curriculum. Although some students who decide on veterinary medicine in the closing years of college are admitted, it is usually wise to make the decision earlier.

By the time students have finished two years of college-level, pre-veterinary studies, they are usually either considering applying to colleges of veterinary medicine or have developed other career choices.

The Veterinary Medical College Application Service

A look at the website of the Veterinary Medical College Application Service (VMCAS), www.vmcas.aavmc.org, provides insight into the application process and the details required on the electronic application. The application format is updated annually and released in June of each year. Completed applications must be submitted in early October to be considered for classes that enter in the fall of the following year.

Beginning in June 2008, all VMCAS applications and accompanying information, including letters of recommendation, must be submitted electronically. That procedure is described in chapter four and its details are available at www.aavmc.org. The long-term process of preparation for applying for admission to veterinary colleges should begin well before that.

Hints for Applicants

As soon as veterinary medicine becomes your career of choice, begin preparing for application. This preparation begins with a personal overhaul as described in this chapter. Also, while still in high school, begin thinking about the colleges to which you could potentially apply to fulfill your pre-veterinary requirements. Then decide on a college offering the required college courses. This means that in high school and in your first college years you must carefully examine the VMCAS website to help determine your college pre-veterinary course selections. The degree to which you can comply with these suggestions will help determine the strength of your application, the nature of required letters of recommendation, and verbal commentary that will surface when your application is finally submitted.

When you are reviewing the VMCAS website, it will become evident that you must start working on the veterinary college applications long before their due date to submit them several weeks before the deadline, which is usually in early October, almost a year before classes start in the following August or September.

Plan on being completely candid in all the information in your application and meticulously detailed in answering the application questions about your experiences and achievements. Admission committees have unique skills for verification of information.

If you are not admitted on your first application, don't be discouraged and be sure to try again.

Summarizing the Preparation for Application

The attitudes, actions, and activities in preparation for application to veterinary colleges that are described above may sound unrealistically overwhelming. The application process requires considerable academic and personal preparation which ideally begins with study and learning habits developed before entering college.

Youth who develop a passion for veterinary medicine can be compared to kids who set an early goal to excel at music, a sport, or as a writer with hopes of becoming a successful professional. They fanatically focus, practice, read, and watch. They usually have some rewarding experience, particularly if supported and encouraged by their parents or guardians. Regardless of the final outcome, these students are better off for the experience. Many of them actually make it.

CHAPTER 4

THE APPLICATION PROCEDURE

Introduction

The procedures and prerequisites for application vary slightly among the 28 US veterinary colleges and the multiple foreign schools to which aspiring Americans apply.

They all require credible scores on standardized tests and from two to four years of pre-veterinary college-level training involving basic sciences and courses in general education.

The application procedure for colleges of veterinary medicine is complicated. It requires thought and effort. Most US colleges use the Veterinary Medical College Application Service (VMCAS) that is managed by the Association of American Veterinary Medical Colleges (AAVMC). It is described below. Applications must be mailed several weeks prior to the submission deadline date. Thus, applicants must get to work as soon as the admission material becomes available.

Each veterinary college requires slightly different college-level courses to be completed before submitting an application. Many colleges and state universities offer pre-veterinary studies as a major. These programs guide students into programs that meet the entrance requirements of regional veterinary colleges and provide the opportunity to bond with like-minded colleagues. However, veterinary colleges accept many applicants who were not involved in formal pre-veterinary programs as long as they meet all their admission requirements.

As mentioned earlier, veterinary colleges in the larger and more populated states have more applicants than those in less populous states. If you are a resident of a state that has a college of veterinary medicine, it is advisable to seek admission in your home state—where your chances are best—as well as in several other states.

Veterinary colleges are continuously changing their admission programs and procedures. Therefore be cautious about seeking advice regarding the requirements of colleges from people who are not currently involved with the institutions.

The changing academic programs and curriculums within each veterinary college are probably irrelevant to applicants because the things that they consider important to their specific career goals are likely to change before their veterinary educations and early professional experiences are completed. These career changes justify the requirements of colleges to include a wide variety of subjects in their required curriculums.

Admission Requirements

The admission brochures and catalogues of each veterinary college outline programs, and VMCAS spells out the specific prerequisite college courses required by applicants. Most of this information can be obtained online from the colleges or from VMCAS at www.vmcas.aavmc.org.

Admission requirements vary but they usually include a broad background in general college education and courses in chemistry, biochemistry, biology, English, and zoology. Some schools expect that applicants will have passed college-level courses in computer science, animal husbandry, microbiology, physiology, physics, or statistics.

The occasional requirements for animal husbandry or animal science courses make it reasonable for potential applicants to do their pre-veterinary work at a university with a college of agriculture. Most veterinary colleges are located at state universities that have colleges of agriculture. These are usually at state-supported institutions and usually—for state residents—have lower tuition and fees than private colleges. This does not exclude high-ranked private colleges from serving as excellent launching pads to veterinary medicine.

Veterinary Technology As an Alternative

If hesitant or otherwise reluctant to study veterinary medicine, students can consider becoming a veterinary assistant, a veterinary technician, or a veterinary technologist. These positions permit hands-on work with animals but require less theoretical and scientific training than the DVM or VMD degrees.

Veterinary technician training is available in most states. Details on careers in veterinary technology and training programs are available from the National Association of Veterinary Technologists in America (NAVTA), which can be reached at www.navta.net/about/state_rep.php. Information on veterinary technology can also be obtained from the American Veterinary Medical Association (AVMA), which is reached on the Internet at http://avma.org/education/cvea.

The Backgrounds of Applicants

Most veterinary schools examine applicants' reasons for seeking a veterinary career. They also look into their other interests. Admission committees will review applicants' extracurricular activities, nonacademic accomplishments and experiences, and their unique individual talents—such as art, music, sports, foreign language skills, or international experience. Many require an essay explaining the applicant's interest in the profession.

In addition, they also look at letters of recommendation and seek evidence of conscientious efforts to achieve academic integrity and personal credibility.

Most veterinary classes have a variety of members including one or more students who already have a master's or doctorate degree.

Selection Procedures

The percentage of applicants admitted is not high and varies from college to college and from year to year. Most prospective students apply to several veterinary colleges. They base their selection on their geographic proximity, the estimated costs, and rumors about the ease of admission. Most applicants have given some thought to at least one alternative career goal.

Admission committees gather information from the responses to questions on the admission application forms, from the required essays that accompany application forms, from verbal and written recommendations, and sometimes from interviews.

Most colleges of veterinary medicine select students with varying professional goals and seek a class with diversity regarding race, gender, geographic origin, age, and military or other life experiences. They seek students who will eventually serve in a variety of professional roles.

Admission Interviews

Each college of veterinary medicine has slightly different criteria for student selection. These change over the years as admission committees rotate within the faculty and as the makeup of the curriculum and student body changes.

Some veterinary colleges interview the top 200 or more applicants and examine their interpersonal skills and their actual understanding of the experiences they have outlined on their application form or in their essay. Occasionally, interviews reveal discrepancies between written information in the application and actual experience or knowledge. Interviews take considerable time and preparation.

Admission committee members, who are usually faculty members with multiple duties, carefully study the applications of the candidates, to phrase questions appropriate to the background and experience of each interviewee. Most admission committee members must be present for the interviews to be effective. For these reasons, many veterinary colleges have given up interviewing applicants.

Periodically, schools that don't interview applicants are urged to do so. Debates on the pros and cons of interviews can be heated. The argument eventually boils down to the issues of weighing advantages of meeting applicants personally and detecting a few major character flaws as opposed to the tremendous investment in faculty time which interviews require. The time involved is usually the winner.

The advantages of interviews are that the committee meet applicants individually and can evaluate their interpersonal styles, professional attitudes, and communication skills. In quizzing candidates on their animal experience or familiarity with the realities of the profession, committee members can get a glimpse of their sincerity and determination. A candidate who has lied on the application is occasionally uncovered at an interview and this disconcerting realization is adequate for rejection because personal integrity is essential for success as a veterinarian.

Some advocates of admission interviews feel that evaluation of communication skills and integrity are adequate justification for interviews. Students applying to veterinary schools which require an interview know that if they are not invited to an interview, their chances of admission are small.

The admission committees select enough students to fill their incoming class, plus a handful of alternates to replace accepted candidates who choose to go in other directions. They use a variety of scoring systems to select the candidates who appear to best match their requirements.

The Veterinary Medical College Application Service

Most US colleges of veterinary medicine participate in the Veterinary Medical College Application Service (VMCAS). This process is conducted by the Association of American Veterinary Medical Colleges (AAVMC) and requires that college transcripts and other application information be sent to that organization's office in Washington, DC. A fee is levied for each college to which an application is submitted. VMCAS screens application forms and transcripts to assure that each applicant meets each college's pre-veterinary requirements.

VMCAS offers prospective students an electronic list of veterinary colleges, their required prerequisite courses, their application procedures, and their required timelines. They also provide a checklist for applicants and a transcript request form.

The application form requires extensive information including the applicant's name and address, state of residence, all high schools and colleges attended, all standard test exams taken and scores, as well as veterinary and animal experience, other employment, and prizes and awards received. Providing accurate details of this information requires that applicants begin as early as possible. Colleges that do not utilize the VMCAS system must be contacted directly.

Each veterinary college has slightly different requirements for college-level pre-veterinary courses, essays, or standard test scores. Applicants initially send applications and transcripts for the colleges of their choosing to the VMCAS. The AAVMC then checks to assure that all the requirements of each college have been met and then forwards applications that survive the initial screening to the respective colleges for their admission committees to make the final decision.

Details on this process, the various tuition levels, and the application procedures of individual colleges can be obtained at www.vmcas.aavmc.org.

Repeated Applications

If your initial application is not accepted, try again. Most colleges of veterinary medicine eventually accept many applicants who they initially reject. Some students initially apply after two or three years of college and are not finally accepted until after they have a bachelor's degree or some collegiate graduate education.

Hints for Applicants

As soon as veterinary medicine becomes your career of choice, begin preparing for application. This preparation starts with a personal overhaul as described in chapter three. Also, while still in high school, begin thinking about the colleges to which you could potentially apply to fulfill your pre-veterinary requirements. Then decide on a college offering the required college courses needed for veterinary schools to consider your application. This means that in high school and in your first college years you must carefully examine the VMCAS website to help determine your pre-veterinary college course selections.

It is evident that you must start working on veterinary college applications long before their due date to get them in by the deadline, which is usually almost a year before classes start.

Plan on being completely candid in all the information in your application and meticulously detailed in answering the application questions about your experiences and achievements. Admission committees have unique skills for verification of information.

If you are not admitted on your first application, don't be discouraged and be sure to try again.

CHAPTER 5

VETERINARY CURRICULUMS

Introduction

All colleges of veterinary medicine have similar but slightly different curriculums, with unique schedules and names for courses. They devote different amounts of time to each subject and use a variety of approaches. Their faculty members place differing emphasis on animal species and on clinical, basic science, or research activities.

Veterinary College Curriculums

Most US and Canadian veterinary colleges have intense four-year curriculums. These curriculums vary from school to school depending on their geographic location, the faculty specialists available, the number and nature of animals in the area, the species of animals the college emphasizes, and their research focuses.

It is almost impossible to select a college with the "best" programs in any species or discipline or which emphasizes clinical teaching, basic science teaching, or research, because these activities change frequently and differing opinions will be offered by those who should know.

The First Year

The first year in veterinary college is mostly basic sciences. These include anatomy of major animal species, biochemistry, pharmacology, and physiology. Some schools add a taste of hands-on clinical medicine to the first year. Many so-called basic science courses have both lectures and laboratories.

In the anatomy laboratories, students dissect embalmed cadavers of animals such as dogs, horses, or cattle in order to learn the appearance, location, and structure of body parts and their relationships to one another. Over the years, more and more veterinary colleges have been replacing teaching cadavers with plastic models that are disassembled and reassembled as anatomic teaching devices. Biochemistry, pharmacology, and physiology laboratories vary among colleges. They usually discuss and demonstrate the activities of various bodily components or pharmaceuticals.

The first year is particularly competitive, with professors seeking to impress students with the rigors of the curriculum. The students—many of whom are academically talented and not accustomed to grades less than "A"—are jockeying for recognition and for positions at the top of the class.

These activities are challenging for students admitted with only two to three years of collegiate pre-veterinary work. It can be shocking when they eventually realize that most of their classmates have already had some version of the basic science courses offered in the first year and that some of them have a master's or doctorate degree in subjects that they are experiencing for the first time. Often, one or two students fail out in the first year, for a variety of reasons that usually differ from actual lack of ability.

The first year offers opportunities for students to become familiar with the veterinary campus and faculty members. It also lets them get acquainted with their classmates and share opinions with other aspiring veterinarians. Those students who did their pre-veterinary work at the same university already feel pretty much at home. New arrivals usually need some acclimation.

The Second Year

Generally, the second year expands on the basics and adds aspects of diseases and bodily responses. Most second-year veterinary curriculums include courses in pathology, toxicology, microbiology, and parasitology. These courses describe the agents that cause diseases and how to recognize and identify them. Depending on the professors, these courses often add a touch of real-life veterinary medicine by describing the clinical signs and lesions of some diseases.

Clinical signs differ from symptoms. Symptoms are effects presented verbally to physicians by human patients and signs are changes that are not verbally described by patients but are recognized by physicians or veterinarians. Because animals can't tell where and how badly something hurts, veterinarians deal only with the signs they observe, and veterinary professors lecture about clinical signs as opposed to symptoms. Lesions are tissue and organ changes resulting from diseases or injuries. Some lesions are evident clinically and some are apparent only during surgery or at postmortem examination.

Some professors who have never been in practice may sidestep mentioning the signs and clinical manifestations of diseases, but will usually discuss treatment and prevention of diseases and the interpretation of diagnostic tests.

By the end of the second year, most student competitiveness has slacked off and students have settled in. They know most classmates by their first names and most of them have lost interest in being the top student in the class.

The Third Year

The third year moves toward specific veterinary disciplines such as: medicine, obstetrics, and surgery; specific diseases of large and small animals; veterinary public health; and other topics. The third year goes more deeply into individual diseases and clinical and diagnostic procedures.

In the third year, students rethink some of the reasons they came to veterinary school and their ideas about how to spend their veterinary careers. This begins when they encounter professors who focus on disciplines like radiology, anesthesiology, or surgery. Other faculty members are species specialists who focus exclusively on dogs, cats, cattle, horses, or other animals.

These faculty members often inspire students to think that they might want to follow in their footsteps. These wishes are often generated by the teacher's personality or enthusiasm as much as by their discipline or species specialty.

During the first three years, veterinary students spend most of their time together as a class. This permits them to get to know one another and to bond into lifelong relationships. It also permits them to develop extracurricular programs involving veterinary fraternities, sororities, and clubs.

Veterinary Student Clubs

During the first year, students are offered opportunities to participate in veterinary college clubs that focus on various animal species, clinical and research specialties, or practice opportunities. Most students continue with club activities until they graduate and acquire a familiarity with the many career options offered by the profession.

The clubs usually have elected officers, hold meetings with invited speakers, and have picnics and parties. They also offer opportunities to meet students in other veterinary classes. Most veterinary colleges' student clubs have faculty advisors.

Commonly there are canine, feline, dairy and beef cattle, equine, laboratory animal medicine, small animal surgery, and zoo animal clubs. There are also Student Chapters of the American Veterinary Medical Association (SCAVMA). SCAVMA meetings usually have guest speakers, picnics, and parties. These activities provide opportunities to bond with classmates, focus on areas of special interest, and develop ideas about their ultimate career goals.

Career goals frequently change remarkably in the first 10 to 20 years after graduation. This is one argument for a complete veterinary education rather than permitting students to select and focus on major subjects and neglect other specialties. This concept of specialization resurfaces periodically as veterinary education is discussed and modified.

The Fourth Year

In the fourth year of veterinary school, students are assigned to clinical rotations in groups of from three to eight students. These clinical rotations provide hands-on experience in small or large animal clinics, clinical pathology or diagnostic laboratories, postmortem facilities, or in ambulatory clinics in which students leave the campus with a faculty member, intern, or resident to treat local farm animals. Some schools provide students with a taste of clinical medicine before senior year but the majority of clinical training occurs in the fourth year of veterinary college.

The fourth year stimulates some veterinary students to reconsider their lifelong reasons for seeking a veterinary career and raises thoughts about species or discipline specializations.

Sometimes the fourth year brings on a major shift in class standing as it moves from the theoretical to more practical hands-on applications, permitting students who may have ranked near the bottom of classes to move rapidly upward as manual dexterity, interpersonal skills, client relationships, and reasoning replace rote memory as measures of excellence.

Toward the end of the fourth year, the almost-veterinarians begin thinking about state and national board examinations that qualify them for licensing. Most states require national board examinations, and some states still require an individual state examination which often necessitates travel to the state for written or practical examinations.

Also, in the fourth year students begin discussing their postgraduation plans. Most have some arrangement to work for a year with a practitioner, often one they have known previously. Most work as assistants to established practitioners but some go into internships or graduate programs, and a few go home to work in a family veterinary practice.

As the last term comes to a close they begin forming car pools for travel to take state board examinations in other states.

Graduation

Graduation from veterinary college is a momentous occasion. The ceremony is usually attended by parents, siblings, spouses, and children of the graduates. Advanced planning is needed to assure availability of nearby motel rooms and dining facilities for each graduate's entourage. The graduation invitations are also announcements that the world has a brand-new veterinarian. They are sent to the graduate's friends, relatives, veterinarians who have helped prepare the new graduate, and to teachers and mentors who have personally provided advice and encouragement that led to the festive occasion.

After receiving their diplomas, the former students are now officially called "Doctor," and embark on a new and exciting phase of their lives. Many will eventually return to academe to pursue further training in various veterinary specialties or to work as faculty members.

Alumni Loyalties

The loyalties of graduates to their colleges of veterinary medicine vary. Many graduates feel extremely grateful for the opportunity to study for the profession. They feel fortunate for the opportunity to join the veterinary community and have a sense of pride about completing a strenuous curriculum. They eagerly anticipate their upcoming careers and look forward to the opportunities to refer challenging cases or clients to the college's clinics and are grateful to their alma mater for providing speakers at veterinary meetings and animal owner organizations. These alums return regularly for reunions and conferences and contribute to scholarship funds and other academic endowments.

A few new graduates will disappear, fade into oblivion, and never be heard from again.

CHAPTER 6
VARIOUS VETERINARY CAREERS

Introduction

The variety of careers open to graduates of veterinary colleges is astonishing. These multiple options are often unappreciated by students or new graduates whose hearts are set on a lifelong career in a chosen practice type. However, within a few years they sometimes tire of practice routines because their enthusiasm wanes or physical exhaustion sets in. When this occurs, their career plans begin to change.

At some point many veterinarians begin looking beyond private practice, at alternative professional careers or new employment opportunities. Moving into specialty areas can provide a change, a feeling of greater expertise, and more control over personal life than is available as a general practitioner or a species-limited clinician.

A Variety of Career Choices

In addition to general practice, small animal practice, and large animal practice as described in chapter one, there are many other veterinary opportunities. These include specialties that qualify veterinarians for a wide variety of academic, corporate, or governmental positions that have regular hours and offer retirement and health insurance benefits.

Most veterinarians are specialists of some sort and thus are obligated to decline invitations to address issues of which they lack experience or the necessary equipment. Such challenges are addressed by veterinary specialties, which require specific skills and experience. Some of these require additional training via internships, residencies, or graduate programs.

Specialties are usually pursued by veterinarians after several years in practice. The years in practice upgrade their interpersonal skills and provide confidence and maturity that render them employable, versatile, and well suited for a variety of career opportunities. When veterinarians decide to specialize, they have many options. These include species specialties, discipline specialties, or mixtures of the two. Some specialties require special training, narrowly focused experience, and, often, certification by examination.

After qualifying as specialists, most experts participate in veterinary specialty organizations that hold annual meetings and publish technical journals to update members on current developments in their field. The combination of experience and meeting attendance often suffices for designation as a specialist. In some cases, advanced training as a resident, intern, or graduate student is necessary. This means a return to the academic world.

Training for Specialties

Formal training for specialties means staying in college after receiving the DVM or VMD degree or returning after spending time in practice. Internships and residencies are usually low-salaried positions, some of which may lack insurance or retirement benefits.

Internships

Interns work under direct supervision of one or more faculty members in veterinary college hospitals. After working with a mentor for a while, they gradually conduct patient care or diagnostic services on their own and may be assisted by veterinary students. Their supervisors are always close at hand for consultation, and they often check on the patients treated by their interns.

If interns do well, after one or two years they may be promoted to residency status, with increased pay and added responsibility for patient care and student instruction. Many successful interns take their residencies at another institution. This expands their backgrounds and familiarizes them with different procedures and outlooks.

Residencies

Residencies are advanced training periods that follow internships. They usually comprise two years of responsibility that increases as their skills and abilities grow. Residencies are occasionally followed by the offer of a faculty position, but usually residents depart to seek other opportunities when their contract ends.

Graduate Programs

If career-changing veterinarians choose to pursue less clinical, more basic science specialties or research endeavors, they usually enroll in graduate programs to pursue a Master of Science (MS) or a Doctor of Philosophy (PhD) degree.

If a faculty position is their ultimate goal, an advanced degree requiring graduate studies is usually essential. Graduate work is often arranged through individual faculty members whom the aspiring candidate knows personally or to whom they have been referred by an acquaintance. Like residents and interns, most graduate students receive meager salaries and minimum benefits. They are expected to perform activities requiring well over 40 hours per week.

Graduate training usually requires advanced coursework and a research project. If graduate students successfully complete their studies and the research, produce an acceptable thesis, and pass their final examination, they are awarded an MS or a PhD degree. These degrees offer convincing evidence of expertise and provide a passport to the academic community.

Specialty Boards and Colleges

There are specialty boards and groups called specialty colleges that formalize the requirements for specialist status in some veterinary disciplines. These groups offer examinations to award diplomate status and to certify the holder's qualifications to practice their specialties.

Status as a Diplomate or Board Certified Specialist requires a DVM or VMD degree, relevant knowledge, and experience in one or more narrow fields, professional credibility and integrity, clinical or research experience, and, often, technical or scientific publications and an examination.

Diplomate status and board certifications are usually a source of pride to their holders, and these designations are added to the recipient's professional biography, business cards, and letterheads to indicate their extra qualifications.

Some veterinary specialties have several organizations. Closely affiliated veterinarians know which of these organizations have the most rigorous membership requirements and which are the most prestigious.

Practice Specialties

Self-employed or privately practicing veterinary specialists can be species experts, discipline experts, or combinations thereof. These specialists are obligated to keep up with advances in their chosen field. Specialists can stay up-to-date with contemporary wisdom more easily than general practitioners, who must know everything about all species and all disciplines.

Discipline and Species Specialists

There are veterinary discipline specialists and species experts. Many professionals combine the two.

Discipline specialists deal with multiple species, utilizing focused diagnostic or therapeutic procedures in areas such as anesthesiology, dermatology, ophthalmology, pathology, surgery, pharmacology, or radiology. This focus permits intense comprehension and enables them to keep up with scientific findings in a narrow field.

Discipline experts serve as consultants and see patients recommended to them by colleagues. They also perform surgery and interpret diagnostic tests and X-rays. Most discipline specialties let veterinarians sidestep emergency situations and allow for some rest on weekends and holidays. Many discipline specialists practice privately, and others work in veterinary colleges or are employed by government agencies or corporations.

Species specialists have a slightly different situation. They are expected to handle all problems of their chosen species. Some animal species specialties include avian, bovine, equine, feline, small ruminant, or swine medicine. Some veterinarians also specialize in aquatic animals, laboratory animals, or zoo animals.

Species-specific specialties are the purview of private, academic, and occasionally, corporate or government veterinarians who conduct health programs for one or more species of animals.

Specialist Organizations

Both the discipline specialists and the species specialists can keep in touch with their area of interest and expertise through their specialty organizations. These associations have annual meetings to discuss emerging issues in their field and they publish journals so members can read focused material on their specialty. Most veterinary specialists are active in these specialty organizations and usually attend local or national meetings. Some specialty organizations have rigorous membership requirements that involve formal training, and some have examinations for membership. Other specialty organizations are less rigorous in their membership requirements. Specialists who are active in specialty organizations often gain reputations, speaking invitations, added income, and prestige beyond that achieved by simply focusing on a certain discipline or species. Specialist organizations vary in size and membership requirements.

The American Association of Bovine Practitioners (AABP) is a relaxed and highly productive specialist organization which is accessible simply by paying annual dues. It publishes a quarterly journal known as *The Bovine Practitioner* and has a widely attended annual meeting that updates members on current information. All members—including those who do not attend the meetings—receive proceedings books that summarize the topics covered at the annual conventions.

The American College of Laboratory Animal Medicine (ACLAM) is an organization with rigorous membership requirements. It works to advance the humane care and responsible use of animals in research. It certifies specialists based on their education and professional experience.

Candidates for ACLAM board certification must pass an examination. In order to qualify to take the examination, they must complete two or more years of carefully monitored post-DVM training, or document at least six years of full-time experience with laboratory animals after receipt of the veterinary degree. Other specialty organizations are described in chapters seven through ten.

Employment in Academe, Government, or Industry

Many academic, governmental, or industrial veterinarians accept their jobs after 3 to 15 years in practice. Only then do they appreciate the differences in the practical, political, and financial environments between private practice and being an employee.

In small private practices, veterinarians are pretty much on their own to choose preferred activities, schedules, and make financial decisions regarding retirement and insurance programs.

Once employed by an organization, veterinarians usually have these decisions made for them, and insurance and retirement benefits are often deducted from salary payments. Employment in academe, government, or industry is very different from private practice. Each of these careers has its own unique advantages.

Academic Careers

Academic careers can involve both species specialties and disciplinary specialties. They are practiced in departments of veterinary science within colleges of agriculture or at colleges of veterinary medicine. They are unique because they permit unusual freedom of professional activity.

Some academic careers—usually teaching or research—require MS or PhD degrees in addition to the DVM. Others require internship or residency experience and specialty board certification. The laws of academic freedom allow academicians to plot their own courses once they obtain tenure.

Tenure implies a permanent position without release except for major infractions. It is awarded after five or more years of satisfactory academic performance. Tenure appointments usually require publication in professional journals.

Sometimes, superb speakers, teachers, clinicians, or individuals involved in delivering information to the public via outreach programs have trouble gaining tenure due to lack of scientific publications or because of administrative priorities. Some academicians with nontenured appointments in areas such as diagnostic laboratories, patient care, and extension positions are eventually awarded tenure, but others are retained on nontenured appointments.

Nontenured academic appointees are usually fully aware that in times of budget crunch, they may be released while less effective but tenured faculty are retained. This uncertainty can make nontenured-track academic positions precarious and forces capable people to leave the academic community. For this reason, the tenure system periodically comes under criticism.

Tenure was devised to preserve academic freedom and protect the rights of faculty to discuss new or controversial issues which may not necessarily express the views of their superiors. Tenure also permits criticism of administrators and institutional systems.

In recent years, the capacity to generate "overhead" dollars accompanying grants and contracts has quietly slipped into tenure requirements at some institutions. Overhead funds help universities cover the added infrastructural costs generated by employees performing research projects funded by grants or contracts. Major research universities receive considerable federal monies for operating expenses in the form of grant overhead. This may partly account for the emphasis on research at some institutions.

When changing jobs, tenured academicians are usually hired with tenure at their new location. Many tenured faculty members insist on tenure appointments when being recruited by another university. Many universities consider tenured faculty from other universities as qualified for immediate tenured appointments.

If offered jobs as deans or department chairs, most faculty members make tenure appointment a requirement for accepting the administrative position. This provides protection against firing for political reasons. While their administrative position can be taken away, they still retain a tenure appointment for other positions in the veterinary college or at the university.

Veterinary colleges train clinical specialists. Many of them refuse to accept a nontenured-track position and sometimes choose to establish private practices close to universities. In these locations, they compete for clientele and patients that the veterinary colleges need for training students, residents, and interns and for supporting their teaching hospitals.

Academic and other veterinary specialists are divided into species-oriented and discipline-oriented endeavors. The species-oriented specialties are described in chapters seven through nine. The discipline specialties are detailed in chapter ten.

Corporate Careers

Corporate careers in veterinary medicine involve employment with pet food manufacturers, drug and pharmaceutical companies, and a variety of other industries. They can be very rewarding. They require loyalty to the employing organization and enthusiasm for their products. Corporate careers usually provide higher incomes than academic or governmental jobs, but there are exceptions to this generalization. These careers can involve veterinary practice, research, sales, administrative, or public relations positions.

Corporate careers are usually more demanding and create higher pressure than academic and governmental careers. Employees of corporations are more closely supervised and more likely to be released for minor divergences from organizational policy. However, like academic organizations and governments, corporations sometimes keep errant employees and shift them with "sideward promotions" when they are functioning ineffectively, rather than undergoing the hassle of firing them and having them institute a lawsuit or spend a lifetime badmouthing their former employers.

Government Careers

Many veterinarians work for state or federal governments. They develop and enforce regulations about animal control, food safety, meat inspection, public health, emergency response activities, and securing borders from entrance of animal diseases or animal-borne human diseases. Each state has individual methods of handling employment of veterinarians and most government agencies have a tenure-like system for retaining employees.

These systems vary in their methodology. Some states offer a two-to-three-year contact that must be renewed upon expiration. In some governmental agencies if an employee is not disciplined or fired in the first one or two years, it takes a major indiscretion to cause them to be released.

Sometimes when government employees are performing below expectations or badmouthing agency policies, they are simply moved via "sideward promotions," to another job to get them out of sight. This rotation process can continue throughout a person's career. Because of complications, possible lawsuits, grievances, or accusations of discrimination, some government agencies are reluctant to fire anyone who has not actually been convicted of illegal activity.

Military Careers for Veterinarians

Few people realize that many veterinarians serve as officers in the Army, where they perform specialized functions. Over the years, thousands of veterinarians have completed the Reserve Officers' Training Corps (ROTC) programs while in college. Then after fulfilling their two-year military obligation in the United States Army Veterinary Corps, many return to civilian life while others remain for lifelong military careers.

The **US Army Veterinary Corps** has about 700 veterinarians and about 1,800 enlisted personnel. The Corps provides for the safety of food for US military personnel stationed abroad. It also provides care for military working dogs and ceremonial horses for the Army, Navy, Air Force, and Marine Corps, and for working animals of the Department of Homeland Security. These animals, mostly dogs, respond to natural disasters and emergencies and work to detect bombs and drugs on land.

Marine mammals (dolphins and sea lions) are trained and cared for by the US Navy Marine Animal Health Program that is staffed by veterinarians from the Army Veterinary Corps. These marine mammals patrol the seas and conduct underwater explorations to detect mines or explosives. They also recover lost objects. The Veterinary Corps also cares for pets of military families that live on military bases. More information can be found at www.veterinaryservice.army.mil.

Except for rare exceptions, most veterinarians employed by government agencies perform effectively and are a credit to the profession. They insert unique perspectives into their military, regulatory, and animal care operations.

Conclusions about Veterinary Careers

Veterinarians specializing in one or more species are sometimes queried about disciplines or species in which they lack a comfortable level of experience, and must confess inadequate knowledge. General practitioners, however, are often expected to know everything about all animal species and all veterinary disciplines.

Veterinarians, be they teachers or corporate or government employees, cannot be experts in each and every discipline. They must often call upon species or discipline specialists, who are discussed in chapters seven through ten.

Few people realize the multiplicity of activities in which veterinarians participate. Students and newly graduated veterinarians don't always consider these specialties as their future careers. It is believed that many more such employment opportunities are available than there are veterinarians willing to fill them.

Fields identified as experiencing a shortage of veterinarians are food animal practice and a variety of regulatory activities such as food safety, public health, and border security. Some experts feel there will soon be shortages of small animal clinicians and most species and discipline specialists.

There are many non-practice veterinary employees of government, industry, academe, and various organizations. These non-private specialists serve the interests of their employing industries and governments, and usually focus on single subjects.

Such positions allow for more night and weekend relaxation time, present less stressful or urgent situations, and provide insurance and retirement benefits. Overall, they are more relaxing than private practices in which owners have full authority and responsibility.

Corporate opportunities usually require practical or other real-world experience. New graduates are rarely hired by corporations, which frequently employ veterinarians with 10 to 15 years' experience in private practice or academe.

The wide variety of available veterinary careers makes the profession suited to individuals with all types of personalities, interpersonal skills, and employment preferences.

CHAPTER 7

CAREERS WITH COMPANION ANIMALS

Introduction

Companion animals are mostly dogs and cats, but there are increasing numbers of people who have pet birds, rabbits, mice, gerbils, and a variety of other species. For the most part, when these pets sicken they are taken to small animal practitioners who apply their professional skills to address the problems of many species.

Some small animal practitioners develop interest and expertise in birds and other less common companion animals and attend lectures on the diagnosis and treatment of their diseases. The reputations of these veterinarians for interest in these species can spread within communities. Some veterinary colleges offer elective courses in diseases of birds, rodents, and various other species that are kept as pets.

All animals share many diseases that require veterinary attention, but each species has some unique medical conditions. These include infectious diseases (some of which are preventable by vaccination), animal emergencies, noninfectious disorders, and a variety of surgical procedures.

Species Specialties

Although most small animal practitioners work with both dogs and cats, some focus on a single species. These species specialists are expected to handle all problems of their chosen animal type. They keep in touch with their area of expertise through specialty organizations which hold annual meetings to discuss emerging issues affecting each animal species.

These organizations publish journals so members can read about issues facing their chosen species. The American Associations of Canine and Feline Practice both have members that can claim species specialist status without specific post-DVM training or passing examinations for board certification.

In addition, there are specialty boards and specialty colleges that require internships, residencies, and/or examinations for board certification as specialists. Some of these boards require periodic reexamination to retain certification status.

Species Specialty Practices

Self-employed or privately practicing veterinary specialists are often experts in the diseases of one or more animal species. They can also be experts in disciplines (see chapter ten) or combinations of species and discipline specialties. The species experts are obligated to keep up with advances that relate to their chosen animal species.

Most species have unique infectious diseases for which vaccinations are available. Species specialists are familiar with the uses, indications, contraindications, and the hazards of each vaccine.

Canine medicine and feline medicine share some common challenges but also have many differences. Some commonalities involve preventative practices like parasite control and vaccinations. There is a need to convince clients of the essential nature of vaccination against numerous infectious diseases which most pet owners are not familiar with. Vaccination not only protects the inoculated animals but lowers the prevalence of the infection so the likelihood of transmission to other animals is reduced. Widespread vaccination partly explains the scarcity of many diseases of dogs and cats in the United States.

Canine Medicine

Because most veterinary students are inspired by the love of pets and by observing veterinarians handle them, small animal medicine is the most common form of veterinary practice in the United States. A significant portion of small animal practice comprises canine medicine. Canine medicine requires a love of dogs, a variety of skills, and continual learning as new diseases and treatments are discovered. Thus, ever-expanding knowledge and experience is required. Most canine practitioners are truly experts, and some are board certified in canine medicine.

Canine practice involves many routine nonemergency medical activities and routine surgical procedures. It also involves emergency medicine and surgery.

Routine Nonemergency Canine Medical Procedures

Routine nonemergency canine medical procedures include vaccinations, the treatment of impacted anal sacs, ear infections, numerous skin conditions, behavioral problems, minor injuries, and a variety of cancers.

Canine Vaccinations

The most common dog vaccinations are administered to prevent rabies, canine distemper, canine hepatitis, canine adenovirus infections, and leptospirosis. Practitioners recommend these products depending on each animal's previous vaccination history, its potential for exposure to wildlife or other dogs, the diseases present in the area, and state regulations and licensing requirements.

Rabies is a usually fatal, bite-transmitted viral infection that affects all mammals including humans. It produces a variety of neurologic disorders in cats, dogs, cattle, horses, small ruminants, and wild mammals. Before dying, infected animals experience behavioral changes and often attack and bite people or other animals. Rabies-infected wild animals may enter inhabited areas which they usually avoid and often develop unprovoked rage, furiously attacking people and other animals.

In the US, skunks, foxes, raccoons, and bats are major reservoirs of rabies. They infect pets by injecting virus-infected saliva with bites. Cats and dogs can infect humans by the same route.

Rabies should be suspected in any dog or cat showing unusual behavior or signs of central nervous disorders. Extreme caution is essential when examining such patients and veterinarians bitten by neurologically disturbed patients must immediately seek medical help, warn its owners, and confine the suspect animal. If the animal dies, they must obtain a laboratory test for rabies on its brain. Most veterinarians have been vaccinated against rabies and they recommend that all cats and dogs receive rabies shots. This high level of vaccination has considerably reduced the incidence of rabies in the United States.

Canine distemper is a highly contagious viral infection of dogs. It causes fever, loss of appetite, runny nose, ocular discharge, and a variety of other disorders including a sometimes fatal nervous sequel that may follow apparent recovery. Vaccination has greatly reduced the incidence of canine distemper.

Infectious canine hepatitis is a viral infection of the canine liver. It causes an elevated temperature, depression, and loss of appetite. Often an opacity (whitening) of the cornea of one eye occurs about a week after the onset of the disease. Hepatitis vaccination usually accompanies distemper shots and has reduced the incidence of the disease.

Canine parvovirus often causes minimal observable signs, but infections in puppies can induce vomiting and a diarrhea which can be fatal. Heart infections can occur in young puppies if the pup's mother was not immunized.

Canine leptospirosis is an infection with one of many types of spiral-shaped organisms, called *Leptospira*, which can infect the urinary tracts of most animals and humans. It is acquired by contact with infected urine. Infected animals show a variety of clinical signs that range from a mild, unobserved infection to an acute febrile disease with occasionally fatal kidney and liver involvement. Leptospirosis vaccines must be repeated frequently.

Nonemergency Canine Conditions

Diseases routinely treated by canine practitioners include a variety of nonemergency afflictions including impacted anal sacs, ear infections, skin conditions, behavioral problems, minor injuries, and a variety of cancers.

Impacted anal sacs are a relatively common canine problem. The anal sacs are small secretory glands located on each side of a dog's posterior opening. They frequently become infected or impacted. The anal sacs are always examined during routine physical examinations, and are routinely expressed by gentle pressure when necessary. If anal sacs become badly infected or impacted, dogs may show pain on defecation, lick at their hind ends, or scrape their bottoms along the ground. Anal sacs also can be treated by application of antibacterial ointments. Sometimes they must be removed surgically.

Ear infections are common in dogs with floppy ears. Dogs' ears must be examined at each visit and carefully cleaned. If excessive wax or infections are present they can be treated with special antibiotic ointments. If the problem persists, surgery to open the ear canal may be required to permit drainage.

Skin conditions of dogs include ringworm, mange, parasite infestations, and a variety of causes for hair loss. The specific cause of skin problems is determined by careful examination of the entire skin, combing and searching for fleas, ticks, mites, or lice, and by microscopic examination of skin scrapings for evidence of fungi, parasites, or infections. Canine dermatology is complicated and skin ailments frequently require prolonged therapy. Parasite control programs are vital to general health as well as to skin conditions.

Behavioral problems in dogs are expressed in various ways and often involve refusal to accept training by their owners. Some behavioral problems include urinating or defecating indoors, eating garbage or feces, biting, excessive barking, jumping on people, aggressive behavior toward other dogs, and sniffing people's genitals.

These behaviors can be addressed by taking them to training classes at an early age, or by consultations with veterinary practitioners or animal behavior specialists.

Minor injuries that don't require surgery can often be treated in the office with a few stitches, a bandage, or a cast. With injuries that have been sutured or bandaged, and also with skin conditions, it is essential to keep dogs from biting at the problem area. This sometimes requires a plastic collar that extends forward to cover the mouth and prevents access of the teeth to body parts. Wound infections can be reduced by antibacterial preparations.

Canine cancers are numerous and increase with age. Those that are visible externally include skin cancers and mammary tumors which can be removed surgically. Cancers of internal organs require X-rays and other diagnostic procedures to learn their location, and biopsies to determine their nature. Like human cancers, canine tumors are challenging to treat and can sometimes result in death.

Canine Emergencies

Canine emergencies come in a variety of forms. Common emergencies involve blood loss, unconsciousness, fractures, or other injuries resulting from automobile accidents, gunshots, or dogfights. These conditions all require immediate attention and some terminate fatally. Their treatment varies with the condition and usually requires prompt application of appropriate surgical procedures and medications as well as prolonged follow-up activities.

Feline Medicine

There is a growing trend among small animal practitioners to specialize in feline medicine. Cats now outnumber dogs in the United States and more and more cat clinics are opening. They seem to be positively addressing a rapidly growing need and they permit practitioners to stay abreast of new information in their field. Some clients prefer to take their cats to species-oriented specialists.

Like canine medicine, feline medicine involves vaccination against infectious diseases, nonemergency medical procedures, emergency medicine, and a variety of diagnostic and surgical methodologies.

Feline Vaccinations

Feline vaccines are available for rabies, feline pneumonitis, feline panleukopenia, feline infectious peritonitis and pleuritis, feline leukopenia, and feline leukemia. Vaccination of cats is an essential part of their health programs. Cat vaccinations should be repeated at recommended intervals. Many feline vaccines are highly effective, but none are perfect. Some feline diseases requiring prevention by vaccination are discussed below.

Rabies in cats is more common than in dogs in the USA. As in other species, this bite-transmitted and usually fatal zoonotic disease causes a variety of neurological manifestations which can result in unprovoked attacks on people and other animals.

Feline pneumonitis is caused by chlamydial infections and usually results in infection in the eyes and upper respiratory tract, mostly involving the nasal passages, nasal sinuses, and the throat. It causes ocular discharge and a runny nose. Treatment with antibiotics is usually successful.

Feline panleukopenia, also known as feline distemper, is a globally distributed viral disease of cats which frequently goes unobserved. It is relatively uncommon in areas where vaccination is practiced. Natural infections can be mild and unnoticed, but it can be fatal for kittens.

Clinical cases are characterized by depression, elevated temperature, a drop in white blood cell counts, ocular and nasal discharges, and inflammation of the oral mucosa. Sometimes, infected cats experience vomiting or sit by their water bowls without drinking.

Feline infectious peritonitis and pleuritis, also known as feline coronaviral vasculitis, usually attacks cats under two years of age. The infection is very common throughout the world. Most infected cats don't sicken but merely develop immunity from the infection. Those that develop the clinical disease may have fever, runny eyes, respiratory distress, or diarrhea. They sometimes develop an accumulation of fluid in the stomach cavity and die.

Feline leukopenia is caused by a tumor-inducing virus that manifests in a variety of ways including elevated temperature and a reduction of immune responses to infections. A vaccine that is administered to young cats is usually effective if given prior to initial exposure to the virus.

Feline leukemia, also called feline lymphoma and leukemia, is a globally distributed, cancer-inducing virus which produces a wide variety of immunological, blood, and cancerous disorders that are often unresponsive to currently available therapies. Vaccination is not always successful.

Nonemergency Feline Medical Procedures

The many nonemergency feline conditions that are treated by veterinarians include behavioral problems, constipation, parasites, skin conditions, and urinary obstructions.

Behavioral problems are relatively common in cats. They have a variety of manifestations including failure to use the litter box (sometimes selecting a favorite couch or rug on which to urinate); aggressive, quarrelsome, or hostile actions; fighting; excessive self-grooming; or continuous twitching. Some of these problems are caused by stress or obsessive-compulsive disorders.

Constipation is a common ailment of cats. It can have numerous causes including lack of available water, inadequate water consumption, injuries or tumors of the intestines, dietary disturbances, and hairballs. Constipation is evident when a cat strains to defecate or by the presence of rock-hard feces in the litter box.

Hard fecal matter is identified by gentle palpation of the abdominal cavity—which may require general anesthesia. It is relieved with enemas, laxatives, lubricants, and occasionally requires surgery.

Parasites of cats include external parasites, also called ectoparasites, and internal parasites (endoparasites). Most feline skin conditions are caused by external parasites which include a variety of mites, ticks, fleas, and fungi, some of which are transmissible to humans and most of which are treatable with insecticide dips or oral medications.

Mites cause contagious mange and hair loss by burrowing into the outer layers of the skin. Ticks and fleas both suck blood from their hosts. Adult ticks and fleas are visible when the hair is closely examined or when the cat is carefully groomed. Feline ringworm is mostly caused by a fungus called *Microsporum canis*, which produces crusty areas of hair loss. Various treatments are available for mange, ringworm, ticks, and fleas.

Endoparasites of cats are numerous and mostly are due to worms and other organisms that infest the gastrointestinal tract and some other locations. Most have one or more intermediate hosts. Endoparasites cause a variety of disorders that include loss of weight and condition, diarrhea, and, sometimes, delayed growth of kittens. Adult worms are sometimes found in feces or vomitus and their eggs are identified by microscopic examination of feces.

Urinary obstructions are common in both male and female cats. While a variety of obstructions develop at various locations in the urinary tract, a common condition is a blockage of the urethra with urinary calculi (stones) or gelatinous plugs that prevent the affected cat from eliminating urine.

The owner may notice blood in the urine, painful urination, and frequent efforts to urinate. Upon examination, the bladder may be distended, and painful upon palpation (gentle touching during physical examination). These obstructions can often be corrected by gentle hydraulic pressure or suction in the urethra. Some calculi require surgical removal.

Feline Emergencies

Feline emergencies include auto accidents, and fractures, cuts, dystocias (difficult or abnormal births), and other injuries.

Auto accidents can be fatal for cats. Those that survive require a variety of manipulative and surgical repairs. Many survive if given prompt attention.

Fractures and cuts from causes other than auto accidents can often be repaired with a few stitches or an appropriately applied cast.

Feline dystocias are relatively uncommon but veterinary care is required if cats are in active, strenuous labor without a delivery for over two or three hours. Veterinarians can relieve most dystocias by careful manual manipulation with sterilized, gloved hands. A caesarian section is occasionally required.

More information about feline medicine can be obtained from the website of the American Association of Feline Practitioners at www.aafponline.org.

Cat Population Control

Many veterinarians are involved in feline population control programs. Because cats have few natural predators and reproduce rapidly, the spaying of female and neutering of male cats is an ever increasing measure to prevent reproduction and help reduce excess cat populations. Feline overpopulations have traditionally been controlled by euthanasia, or "putting down" thousands of stray or unwanted cats.

This mass euthanasia trend is being addressed by a variety of pet adoption organizations that require adopted cats to be neutered. Such programs will help prevent the US from being overrun by feral cats which can decimate bird populations and hasten the demise of endangered avian species.

Free-roaming cats also provide breeding grounds for multiple pet animal diseases and some human diseases such as rabies. Feral animals, defined as originally domestic creatures that have established wild populations in remote or populated areas, will require ever increasing cooperation between pet adoption agencies and the veterinary profession as human populations invade currently unpopulated areas.

For more information, contact the American Association of Feline Practitioners at www.aafponline.org.

Conclusions about Companion Animal Careers

The future is bright for veterinarians in small animal medicine because of the increasing numbers of dogs and cats and the growing concern their owners have about their pets' well-being.

New techniques and procedures for diagnosis and treatment of companion animal diseases are constantly emerging. Thus, companion animal veterinarians require constant updating. Some authorities are predicting a shortage of companion animal veterinarians as the nation's population grows.

CHAPTER 8

CAREERS WITH FARM ANIMALS AND HORSES

Introduction

Large animal practitioners work with cattle, goats, horses, pigs, and sheep. These practices provide routine and emergency services for their clientele. Large animal veterinarians must be available around the clock unless they are in a group practice or trade days off with nearby colleagues.

Bovine Medicine

Many large animal practitioners deal mainly with beef or dairy cattle. They handle routine nonemergency procedures such as vaccination and pregnancy examinations, and a variety of emergencies. They also oversee herd health programs.

Bovine Vaccinations

Vaccines are available for a variety of cattle diseases present in the US. Vaccines for exotic diseases like foot-and-mouth disease are stockpiled by federal authorities for use in emergencies.

Vaccines for domestic bovine diseases are administered as individual products or in a variety of combinations. They include vaccines to prevent infectious bovine rhinotracheitis, bovine viral diarrhea, bovine myxovirus parainfluenza-3, and leptospira pomona.

Infectious bovine rhinotracheitis (IBR) is a viral infection that produces elevated temperature, respiratory distress, reduced milk production, weight loss, and abortion. IBR-infected cattle can harbor the IBR herpesvirus for life and can shed it during stress-induced reactivations years after their initial infection. IBR vaccines are available individually and in several combinations.

Bovine viral diarrhea (BVD) can cause fever, a sometimes fatal diarrhea, vesicles (blisters) in the mouth, and abortion or congenital defects. Calves born to cows infected during pregnancy can become lifelong carriers of the virus and serve as the source of new infections. BVD vaccines are available individually and in combination with other products.

Bovine myxovirus parainfluenza-3 (BPI-3) is a usually mild viral infection that combines with stress and mixed bacterial infections to produce "shipping fever." This debilitating and sometimes fatal respiratory disease usually occurs in transported or otherwise stressed cattle. BPI-3 vaccines are usually combined with other products.

Leptospira pomona is a thin coiled bacterium that lives in cows' urinary tracts. It causes an acute febrile disease and abortion. Cattle can be vaccinated for leptospirosis alone or in combination with other vaccines. Leptospira pomona can sometimes produce a febrile infection in humans.

Bovine Emergencies

Emergencies that are frequent in dairy and beef cattle include calving difficulties, prolapsed uteruses, acute mastitis, and bloat.

Calving difficulties (technically known as dystocias) require prompt attention to save the life of the calf and minimize damage to its dam (female parent). Most difficult births can be corrected by careful manipulation of the fetus, but some require a caesarian section.

During normal birth, the calf is in an anterior presentation, positioned upright with its front feet extended and the head resting on them. Upon uterine contractions with a widely dilated cervix, the front feet appear and are immediately followed by the head, shoulders, torso, and the hind legs.

If the calf has abnormal size or shape or is in an inappropriate position, the situation requires immediate attention. Farmers will often try to correct abnormal presentations such as when the head or one front leg is bent backward. If their efforts don't provide prompt results, they usually call a veterinarian.

On arrival of the veterinarian, the calf may already be dead. Veterinarians quickly reduce the cow's straining to expedite fetal manipulation and minimize the risk of rupturing the uterus. Uterine relaxation is achieved by intravertebral injection of a local anesthetic into the epidural space that surrounds the spinal cord.

After the anesthetic injection (epidural) is administered, the cow ceases its straining efforts and the fetal position can be safely adjusted. After administering the epidural, veterinarians scrub and sanitize the cow's posterior and their hands and arms before entering the uterus to examine the calf's size, shape, presentation, and position. The birth canal is heavily lubricated before pressure is applied to extract the calf.

If it is a simple dystocia, the calf is safely delivered by attaching obstetrical chains to the front legs and slowly extracting it with firm pressure. If additional pressure is needed, it can be applied with a fetal extractor. The fetal extractor is a five-foot-long bar that fits comfortably behind the thighs of the cow. It has a pulley that permits controlled, steady pressure until the calf is delivered.

Serious presentations or fetal anatomical abnormalities require meticulous rearrangement to achieve safe delivery. These are often handled by a caesarian section if there is a chance of recovering a live calf. If the fetus is already dead, the major concern becomes the health of the dam, and the fetus may be removed by an embryotomy, which involves dissection and removal of the offending parts.

Prolapsed uterus is an often fatal bovine emergency. Sometimes after a normal birth, the uterus inverts and follows the calf into the stall. This uterine protrusion is called a prolapse. Prolapsed uteruses are urgent emergencies because they create interference with circulation and can cause potentially fatal gangrene.

When promptly replaced, prolapsed uteruses have already become heavily contaminated with feces, and can become badly infected, causing metritis (uterine inflammation) which may prevent future pregnancies.

If promptly replaced, many uterine prolapse cases survive. If a farmer calls saying a cow has "cast her withers," veterinarians know it is a prolapse and they drop everything and head for that farm.

Acute mastitis is a frequently occurring, severe inflammation of the milk-producing organ. The term mastitis includes any inflammation of the udder.

The cow's udder, or milk-bag, has four distinctly separate compartments (called quarters). Each is drainable by a large teat through which milk is extracted by the sucking motions of a nursing calf, by the alternate squeezing and relaxing of a farmer's hand, or by milking machines containing four rubber-lined metal tubes which obtain milk by intermittent application and relaxing of gentle suction.

Mild udder inflammation is common. It is evidenced by small white flakes or clots in the milk from the affected quarter. Flakes and clots are distinguishable by a single squirt of milk on black plastic in a strip cup or strip plate and are treatable by inter-mammary injections of mastitis ointments.

Chronic mastitis increases the cell count of the milk and is detected by tests at milk plants. Milk from treated quarters must be withheld from shipment and milk plants can reject an entire milk shipment if drugs are detected in it. Veterinarians and feed stores sell boxes of mastitis tubes which farmers administer to affected quarters after careful cleaning and disinfection of the teat end.

Acute mastitis is a heated inflammation, swelling, and reddening of one or two quarters. It rapidly becomes a generalized infection characterized by fever, rapid respiration, loss of appetite, cessation of milk production, and sometimes death. Careful examination of a cow's udder for flakes, clots, swelling, or heating is a routine step in the physical examination of sick cattle.

Treatment of acute mastitis requires milking out the infected quarter—sometimes assisted by hormone injections—and by intramuscular, intramammary, and intravenous injections of antimicrobials. Despite these efforts, some acute mastitis cases succumb, particularly if they are not detected and treated early.

Bovine bloat is also an emergency. Bloat involves an interference with the regurgitation (belching) mechanism. It often occurs—sometimes on a herd basis—in cattle grazing on rapidly growing legume pastures.

In bloat, the fourth and largest bovine stomach (the rumen) fills with gas and the distension is visible as a balloon-like swelling on the left flank, behind the last rib. If not relieved promptly, it can inhibit breathing and terminate fatally.

Bloat is best relieved by passing a lubricated tube down the esophagus, into the rumen, and letting the gas escape. When this fails or if there are multiple cases present, the rumen pressure can be relieved by puncturing the expanded rumen with a trocar and cannula. A trocar is a sharp, pointed rod that fits into a metal tube (the cannula). Together, they are jammed through the skin into the highest point of the distended rumen. After it is inserted, its pointed central portion (the trocar) is removed, leaving a nonirritating hollow tube (the cannula) through which gas rushes out, relieving the distress.

Ideally the skin should be shaved and disinfected before this procedure but in herd episodes, this detail is often omitted because of the urgency of the situation. Trocar wounds can result in infections, either local abscesses or internal infections of the lining of the stomach cavity. These possibilities are better than the fatal alternative which can result if bloat is left untreated.

Nonemergency Bovine Disorders

The nonemergency calls to treat cattle usually consist of foot rot, acetonemia, retained placenta, hardware disease, and calf scours.

Foot rot is a bacterial infection that causes an accumulation of smelly, rotten material between the claws of a cow's hooves. It causes lameness, lowered milk production, and sometimes loss of appetite. It usually affects one or two of a cow's feet and causes them to limp. During summer months when cows are on pasture or in muddy barnyards, veterinarians treat several lame cows daily.

While some bovine lameness results from cracked hooves or puncture wounds, foot rot is the most common cause of bovine limping. Its treatment requires trimming and examining the foot and—if it is foot rot—removing the necrotic tissue, cleaning and disinfecting the interdigital spaces, bandaging the foot, injecting the cow with antimicrobials, and prescribing that her milk be withheld from the market. Infected cows are kept in the barn (and out of the mud) until the lameness subsides and the interdigital space heals.

Acetonemia, meaning acetone in the blood, is also known as ketosis. It is a metabolic dysfunction of high-producing dairy cows that usually occurs within six weeks of calving. It is characterized by reduced appetite, an uncharacteristic preference for hay rather than grain, and a semisweet breath odor that is easily recognized.

The diagnosis of acetonemia is confirmed by detecting ketones in milk or urine using test kits. It is treated with intravenous injections of a 50% dextrose solution and/or inoculation with steroids.

Retained placenta occurs following calving if the uterine structure that nourishes the fetus is not shed with the calf. Retained placentas hang from the birth canal for days and become heavily contaminated with manure. The dangling placenta provides an expressway for access of fecal-borne microorganisms into the uterus, which is vulnerable to infections. These infections, called metritis, can be debilitating and result in infertility.

Retained placentas—if not dropped within a day or two—were formerly removed manually by veterinarians. This procedure is no longer recommended. The affected cows are now carefully observed and if they sicken or develop a fever, they are treated with antibacterial medications.

Hardware disease, technically called traumatic reticular peritonitis, results when a cow swallows nails, screws, or rusty scraps of fence or baling wire that have been chopped by harvesting equipment. Grazing cows can easily pick up and swallow such objects.

Wires and nails collect in the reticulum, the skullcap-shaped first of the four bovine stomachs. They can lie there for some time. When this pouch contracts during digestion, sharp objects sometimes penetrate its wall, permitting germ-laden intestinal contents to infiltrate tissues. The resulting painful infection causes a cessation of gastrointestinal mobility, fever, and a characteristic humpbacked posture. When diagnosed, hardware can often be alleviated by antibiotic injections or by an operation called a rumenotomy.

In this operation, the surgeon enters the gastrointestinal tract via the rumen, the largest of the four stomachs, through an incision on the cow's left side behind the last rib. After removing a bushel or more of grassy stomach contents the reticulum in front of the rumen is accessed to remove its metal collection, hopefully including the troublemaker that punctured its wall and is the seat of the painful infection.

If the wire has penetrated the diaphragm and the heart sac (the pericardium), it seeds the outer cardiac surface with infectious organisms and the heart is soon surrounded by a sac of pus that reduces its ability to function and eventually causes death. Cows with this fatal condition, called traumatic pericarditis, usually have distended jugular veins, rapid heartbeats, and shortness of breath, and are euthanized.

Calf scours, the common name for diarrhea of young calves, is caused by a variety of infectious agents—mostly bacteria. It can be mild or accompanied by fever, debility, and sometimes death. Most farmers treat mild cases of calf scours with antibiotics and antidiarrheal drugs. When the calves are seriously debilitated or if the condition spreads rapidly, farmers usually call the veterinarian. By that time, it is often too late and some victims have already succumbed.

More information about bovine medicine can be obtained from the American Association of Bovine Practitioners at their website, www.aabp.org.

Equine Medicine

There are light horses, namely riding, saddle, and race horses, and draft (work) horses. The draft horses are bigger, stronger, slower, and less excitable than the light horses. They are used as show animals or to pull wagons and equipment on terrains too slippery for tractors. They are often doctored by general practitioners who visit the farms on which they are kept.

Some equine practitioners specialize in riding horses or race horses. The race horse specialists often maintain two or more residences so they can be present when racetracks open in different climates. Like other species specialists, equine practitioners administer vaccines, treat nonemergency medical issues, and handle emergencies.

Equine Vaccinations

Available equine vaccines include antibacterial vaccines for strangles and numerous vaccines against viral infections.

Strangles is an acute contagious bacterial infection of the lymph nodes in the throat area. It is also known as equine distemper or equine shipping fever. It is caused by *Streptococcus equi* and most commonly occurs among transported horses which have been assembled from various locations.

Horses with strangles have a fever, runny eyes, and severe swellings and abscesses of the throat that cause pain when swallowing. These abscesses occasionally rupture, causing external drainage of pus. Strangles vaccines are available but they are not all totally safe or uniformly effective.

Equine viral infections are preventable by inactivated and modified live virus vaccines that offer varying levels of protection against equine influenza, equine viral arteritis, and the equine herpesviruses. There are also vaccines for Eastern, Western, and Venezuelan viral encephalitis, and West Nile virus.

Equine influenza is a rapidly spreading viral infection characterized by fever, coughing, runny nose, and loss of appetite. It is very debilitating but usually not fatal unless accompanied by secondary bacterial pneumonia. It is partially preventable by a variety of vaccines that are injected intramuscularly or sprayed into the nostrils.

Equine viral arteritis is a viral infection that is frequently mild and unobserved. It often causes fever, depression, runny eyes and nose, and edematous swelling of the hind legs. Swelling also occurs in the udder of females and sex organs of males. It is partially prevented by vaccination, which is not recommended for pregnant mares due to its potential for causing abortion.

Equine herpesviruses cause two syndromes, namely viral rhinopneumonitis and equine viral abortion. They are widespread among horse populations.

Equine viral rhinopneumonitis is a contagious respiratory disease characterized by fever, coughing, nasal discharge, and swelling of the lymph nodes in the throat. It is common in foals.

Equine viral abortion is caused by a different herpesvirus infection, so a separate vaccine is used in attempting its control. Both of these viruses cause lifelong latent infections that can occasionally be reactivated by stress and may spread infections to immunologically naïve horses.

The equine viral encephalitides include Eastern equine viral encephalitis, Western equine encephalomyelitis, Venezuelan equine encephalomyelitis, West Nile virus encephalitis, and numerous variations of each. These viruses are mosquito transmitted and cause depression, fever, swallowing difficulties, walking in circles, impaired vision, erratic wandering, and other neurological disorders. They are frequently fatal and partly preventable by vaccination.

The indications and contraindications of equine vaccines are complicated. Vaccinations must be sorted out depending on the age, use, previous vaccinations, sex, and pregnancy status of each horse as well as the time of year and the geographic location.

Nonemergency Equine Medicine

Nonemergency equine veterinary services address lameness, respiratory diseases, dentistry, parasite control programs, routine physical examinations, and nutritional consultations.

Equine lameness is disruptive to riding, racing, or draft horses and results in frequent calls to veterinarians. Diagnosis of the cause of lameness is challenging. Before proceeding too far, most veterinarians called to treat equine lameness conduct a complete physical exam on the patient to assure that the problem is actually in the legs or feet.

When lifting the horse's leg, the veterinarian checks all joints for problems before cleaning and trimming the hoof to find cracks, punctures, or infections. Unless the condition is acute and painful, walking or trotting on a safe, dry surface can provide clues to the location and nature of the problem. Equine specialists diagnose lameness with physical exams, X-rays, and sometimes with magnetic resonance imaging (MRI). Multiple disorders of the equine hoof and joints are described in *The Merck Veterinary Manual.*[2]

Equine respiratory diseases include the viral infections discussed under vaccination (above) and the secondary bacterial infections that frequently follow them. These require prompt treatment with antibacterial drugs and isolation of affected animals to prevent spread.

Equine dental work is a routine part of equine practice. Horses have more dental problems than most animals due to the anatomy of their jaw, which creates excess tooth grinding and makes for sharpened teeth that can cut the tongue, mouth, and cheeks. These cuts result in bleeding, incomplete chewing of feed, and dropping of partially chewed hay and grain on the ground.

Veterinarians routinely examine horses for sharp teeth and file them with an instrument called a float. Floating teeth is a routine part of equine practice. Dental examination can be done by hand with cooperative and gentle horses, but less cooperative patients require use of a metal mouth brace, called a speculum, to hold the mouth open. Some equine dental work requires general anesthesia.

Parasite control programs are essential for the nutritional efficiency of horses. Intestinal parasites commonly carried by horses include tapeworms, stomach worms, stomach bots (botfly larva), pinworms, and others. Bloodworms can also be present. Each of these can produce unthriftiness (poor growth) and sometimes diarrhea or other problems. They are treatable with a variety of medications called anthelmintics, some of which are not usable on pregnant mares. Because of the number of equine diseases that are mosquito borne, it is advisable to have mosquito control programs in stables.

Routine equine physical exams are common procedures for equine veterinarians. People considering purchasing a horse and those preparing horses for sale, shipment, or shows often require a veterinarian-signed health certificate to accompany them. A similar exam is conducted on horses when they are sick.

When performing a physical examination, the veterinarian checks their skin for signs of ringworm, summer sores, or other afflictions. They also check the temperature, pulse, and respiratory rates to assure they are within normal ranges. They check the heart and lungs with stethoscopes and examine the mouth, nasal passages, and eyes. They usually perform a rectal examination to seek problems with abdominal contents and may conduct a fecal examination for evidence of worm eggs. They examine the leg joints and hooves for abnormalities. Before the health certificate is signed, the gait of the horse is checked as it is walked, trotted, and galloped. Notes are made indicating any possible problems.

Equine nutrition is an occasional contributor to health problems, and nutritional consultations are occasionally requested by horse owners, especially if horses appear unthrifty or are losing weight. The dietary needs of horses vary depending on age, use, stage of pregnancy, and medical condition.

Many horses are adequately nourished solely by grazing on fresh green pastures, with access to water. Grain supplementation is necessary if the horses on pasture are pregnant mares or nursing, are rapidly growing colts, or if the pasture is depleted.

Equine Emergencies

Equine emergencies include dystocia, cuts and wounds, colic, and acute illnesses in foals. They also include injuries, fractures, and lacerations.

Dystocia (difficult birth) is rare in horses, but when it occurs, primary concerns are to deliver a live foal and limit damage to the mare. Newborn foals frequently require procedures to induce normal breathing after a difficult birth. They also occasionally develop blood-borne infections (septicemia) that require treatment with antibacterial drugs.

Cuts and wounds, particularly on the legs of horses, can incapacitate otherwise healthy animals. They need immediate attention due to their susceptibility to infections, which can be painful and result in lameness.

Injuries resulting in fractures and lacerations often require splints, stitches, and immobilization, which is difficult to achieve due to the equine anatomic structure and the impossibly of confining horses to bed rest.

Colic is an acute localized abdominal pain or discomfort caused by obstruction, gas accumulation, or swelling or twisting of gastrointestinal organs in horses. It has a variety of causes. Affected horses demonstrate discomfort by pawing at the ground, kicking at their abdomens, or repeatedly turning to look at their flanks. Many colic cases are extreme medical emergencies.

Colic requires a complete physical examination—including rectal examination—and knowledge of the anatomy and function of the equine digestive system. Considerable skill and wisdom are required to determine the exact location and cause of the disturbance and to determine the specific medical or surgical treatment needed to relieve the pain or save the patient's life. If the colic is severe, it can terminate fatally. The earlier the diagnosis and treatments are initiated, the greater the chances are for recovery.

A wide variety of abdominal disorders are commonly characterized as colic. They are urgent medical emergencies. These can involve intestinal blockage, torsion, or rupture and can be fatal or so serious as to require emergency surgery or euthanasia. Prompt treatment is sometimes successful.

Treatment is often achieved by administration of medicine via a stomach tube. Successful treatment of colic requires systematic examination to determine the location and cause of the problem and usually requires intravenous administration of fluids to restore blood volume and maintain electrolyte balances.

Acute illness in foals is usually considered an emergency. Early in their lives, foals can be affected with a variety of illnesses that appear suddenly. These illnesses include bacterial or viral diarrhea and so-called "heat diarrhea," which occurs in nursing foals when the dam has her first post-foaling estrous. Infectious diarrhea in foals can be relatively mild, but is sometimes fatal so it requires prompt diagnosis and treatment.

Additional information can be obtained from the American Association of Equine Practitioners at www.aaep.org, and the American Horse Council, www.horsecouncil.org.

Small Ruminant (Caprine and Ovine) Medicine

Small ruminant veterinarians specialize in sheep and/or goat medicine. Because sheep and goats are smaller and represent less financial investment than cattle and horses and can be less emotionally cherished by people than dogs and cats, veterinarians are less likely to be called by small ruminant owners than by large animal or pet clients. There are many exceptions to this generalization.

Sheep and goats have many size, nutritional, and management similarities and share many infections, so they are frequently addressed collectively in veterinary texts and college lectures. In suburban and populated areas, sheep and goats must be confined—sometimes at great expense—to prevent them from wandering into traffic, climbing, or being attacked by dogs. However, sheep and goats differ in many ways. Goats are more aggressive and climb more than sheep, and tend to fight and escape captivity more frequently than sheep do.

Infections Shared by Goats and Sheep

Several infections are shared by sheep and goats and they can be addressed under the title of small ruminant medicine. These include contagious ecthyma, caseous lymphadenitis, and brucellosis.

Contagious ecthyma is a viral infection that affects both goats and sheep. It is also called orf or sore mouth. Contagious ecthyma usually affects young sheep and goats by causing a progression of lesions on the lips and sometimes on the skin of the feet.

The lip lesions initially resemble pimples, or papules. They soon become rapidly rupturing blisters that can spread to the udder and teats of females nursing infected offspring. Eventually these lesions scab over, but in the process young sheep and goats can lose weight and condition. Contagious ecthyma can be prevented by vaccination.

Caseous lymphadenitis also affects sheep and goats. It is caused by a bacterium called *Corynebacterium pseudotuberculosis* that is occasionally transmitted to humans. Caseous lymphadenitis produces slow-growing, painful abscesses in lymph nodes and in other parts of the body. When they are visible to the naked eye there is a decline in sale value of affected animals. Control measures include vaccination (approved only for sheep), sanitary measures, and isolation of infected animals.

Brucellosis affects both goats and sheep. In goats it is caused by *Brucella militensis*. Ovine brucellosis is caused by both *B. ovis* and *B. militensis*. In goats brucellosis produces abortion. In sheep it occasionally produces abortion but is best known for producing orchitis (inflammation of the testicles) and epididymitis (inflammation of the epididymis). Both cause male infertility.

Both sheep and goats can be infected with numerous other bacterial and viral infections. Further information is available from the American Association of Small Ruminant Practitioners at www.aasrp.org.

Goat Medicine

Healthy goat populations require responsible management. Goats tend to climb fences and run loose if not adequately confined. They will also climb into feeding troughs and contaminate them with feces, so their herd-mates refuse to eat the contents.

Male goats tend to fight and must be kept apart. They should have their horns removed by a process called debudding, which is usually performed in the first two weeks of life. They are frequently treated for fight wounds that include lacerations, fractures, and eye injuries.

In addition, goats must be treated for lungworms and several gastrointestinal parasitic infestations including coccidiosis and liver flukes. Goats should be vaccinated for contagious ecthyma if it is present in the herd. They also suffer from a bacterially induced problem called clostridial diarrhea.

Goats can be infected with a virus called caprine arthritis and encephalitis virus that causes an unobservable (subclinical) infection or a debilitating arthritis. Effective treatments or vaccines are lacking for caprine arthritis and encephalitis, so the best available control measures involve herd testing and isolation or removal of infected goats.

Goats get mastitis less frequently than cattle do. Caprine mastitis is less obvious and less responsive to treatment than its bovine and ovine counterparts.

Sheep Medicine

Sheep suffer from viral and bacterial diseases, lameness, parasitic infestations, neurological disorders, white muscle disease, mismanagement and nutritional problems, and other medical challenges.

Ovine viral and bacterial infections include sheep pox and a variety of viral and bacterial pneumonias, some of which are contagious and require isolation of infected animals.

Ovine lameness can result from bruising, or from infections, puncture wounds, or fractures. Lameness is often ignored by owners and allowed to heal spontaneously. If the lameness persists indefinitely, the affected animals are sometimes sent to slaughter or treated by veterinarians.

Parasitic infestations are common and important health hazards for sheep. They include a wide variety of intestinal parasites, which can exist at low levels without producing any effects visible to their owners. At increasing levels of infestation, they induce diarrhea, weight loss, and, occasionally, death.

Some ovine intestinal parasites suck blood from their host's gut and cause anemia and edematous swellings under the chin, which are called bottle jaw. Most parasitic infestations are acquired from pastures and pens contaminated with feces that are loaded with worm eggs.

Worm infestations are diagnosed by microscopic examination of their eggs in fecal samples. They are controlled by avoiding overcrowding of pastures and pens and by use of worm medications (anthelmintics). Sheep are also afflicted with lungworms and liver flukes.

Sheep are occasionally infested or bothered by external parasites including lice, flies, bots, and mange-producing mites. These are addressed by environmental hygiene and medication.

Ovine neurological disorders result from scrapie, tumors, parasitism, rabies, trauma, chemical poisonings, or viral infections. Their diagnosis and treatment can be challenging. Most ovine neurological disorders occur sporadically and are best diagnosed by postmortem examinations or laboratory tests.

Scrapie is a neurologic disease of sheep caused by subcellular particles that are smaller than viruses. It results in behavioral changes, twitching, and eventual death. It is believed that feeding of bone meal from scrapie-infected sheep causes bovine spongiform encephalopathy (BSE), a cattle disease transmissible to humans who consume meat or by-products from BSE-infected cattle.

White muscle disease in young sheep and goats is also called stiff lamb disease. It is caused by a deficiency of selenium and vitamin E and it causes parallel bands of whiteness in leg, diaphragm, and heart muscles, stiffness and lameness in the legs, and sometimes death. Many sheep breeders routinely inject their lambs with a selenium compound (sodium selenite) and vitamin E to stave off stiff lamb disease.

Ovine mismanagement and nutritional problems can contribute to parasitic infestation and poor fencing can permit dog attacks and other injuries.

Small Ruminant Emergencies

In sheep and goats, acute mastitis may be fatal if it is not treated promptly. Milder mastitis infections can markedly reduce milk production, slow the growth of lambs and kids, and occasionally induce the death of young animals that are nursing infected dams.

Sheep often develop bacterial or viral pneumonia that requires treatment. Small ruminants can also develop lungworm infestations, which are diagnosed at postmortem examination or by finding worm larvae in the feces. These ailments all require treatment and preventive management practices such as isolation of recently shipped animals, alleviation of crowded housing conditions, and provisions for adequate ventilation and nutrition.

The American Sheep Industry Association (www.sheepusa.org) can provide additional information.

Porcine Medicine

Veterinarians specializing in porcine medicine deal with corporate swine-rearing operations that raise thousands of pigs from farrow to finish, with privately owned swine farms, and with small farmers who raise a few pigs. These vets deal with some diseases that are confined to swine, some diseases that swine share with other animal species, and some human diseases for which swine serve as principal reservoirs.

In pursuing swine medicine, veterinarians must understand and address porcine infectious diseases, a variety of parasites, frequent nutritional and reproductive problems, and health situations arising from breeding, farrowing, nursing, or the environments in which pigs are raised. Like most livestock species, swine are affected by a variety of intestinal diseases caused by bacteria, viruses, and parasites.

Diseases Largely Confined to Swine

Diseases that primarily affect swine are: hog cholera, African swine fever, vesicular exanthema, edema disease, and swine erysipelas.

Hog cholera, also called classical swine fever, is an acute, highly contagious viral disease that is characterized by elevated temperature, loss of appetite, and lesions that vary from reddening of the skin to hemorrhage and purple skin discoloration.

Massive internal hemorrhages are seen on postmortem examination of hog cholera–infected pigs. Hog cholera has been eradicated from the USA, Canada, Australia, and New Zealand and is present in only a few countries.

African swine fever is a highly fatal, exotic porcine viral infection with similarities to hog cholera. The two can be distinguished only by laboratory tests that identify the distinctly different causative viruses. African swine fever is mostly seen in continental Africa where it is maintained by several species of ticks. It has spread to Europe on several occasions. While it resembles hog cholera, it is more rapidly spread and usually more lethal than hog cholera.

Vesicular exanthema is a highly infectious porcine viral infection that produces blisters on the nose, in the mouth, and on the feet. Vesicular exanthema requires laboratory tests to distinguish it from foot-and-mouth disease, vesicular stomatitis, and swine vesicular disease. It is also called San Miguel sea lion disease because the causative virus has been isolated from dying sea lions and seals in the Pacific Ocean.

Edema disease, sometimes called gut edema, is a fast-spreading disease that strikes healthy, rapidly growing pigs soon after weaning. It is caused by several strains of *E. coli* bacteria. Edema disease causes fluid-induced swelling of the head and sometimes paralysis. It has a sudden onset and is often fatal. Treatment with antibiotics is only partly successful. On postmortem examination, the stomach lining is swollen with fluid.

The control and prevention of edema disease involves environmental sanitation, vaccines against the specific but variable *E. coli* strains, and injections of serum antibodies.

Swine erysipelas is an acute bacterial disease that sometimes causes sudden death. Usually, however, it results in stiffness and reluctance to walk, red or dark discoloration of the skin, and sometimes abortion. It responds to early injections of penicillin.

Porcine Involvement in Multispecies Diseases

Some multispecies diseases that affect swine are meliodosis, salmonellosis, porcine tuberculosis, and trichinosis.

Meliodosis is a soil and waterborne disease caused by a bacterium called *Bacillus pseudomallei* (and many other names). It causes abscesses of the skin and internal organs. The infection is difficult to treat and requires prolonged administration of antibiotic combinations which are not always successful. The organisms that cause meliodosis have worldwide distribution, but active infections are extremely rare in the United States.

Salmonellosis, an infection with any of more than a thousand different bacteria of the *Salmonella* species, occurs frequently in swine. The gastrointestinal tract of swine can be silently infected with many salmonella strains, some of which can cause diarrhea or septicemia. *Salmonella choleraesuis* and *Salmonella typhimurium* can be secondary invaders in swine infected with porcine reproductive or respiratory infections. Salmonellosis is a frequent cause of diarrhea outbreaks in swine.

Porcine tuberculosis is usually acquired from poultry, cattle, or humans and can be the result of direct or close contact with *Mycobacterium avium*, *Mycobacterium bovis*, or *Mycobacterium tuberculosis*.

Trichinosis in swine results from infestation with a roundworm named *Trichinella spiralis*, which undergoes a complex life cycle and then forms cysts in the muscles of many carnivorous animals. The infestations in animal hosts are usually not observed. However, human infestations can be serious.

Swine as Reservoirs of Human Diseases

Swine are reservoirs of several human diseases including trichinosis and nipah virus infections.

Human trichinosis is the basis of warnings about eating incompletely cooked pork. The Hebrew exclusion of dietary pork is also based on trichinosis. It is a serious and sometimes fatal human disease marked by fever, difficult breathing, swollen upper eyelids, edema, painful muscular calcification, and, rarely, death.

In man, trichinosis results from invasion by larvae of *Trichinella spiralis* into the muscles and is acquired by eating incompletely cooked pork and, occasionally, rare meat of bears or other wildlife.

Nipah virus disease emerged in Malaysia in the late 1990s. It is transmitted to swine by infected bats. Infected pigs develop fever, respiratory distress, and a cough that inspired the name "barking pig syndrome." Occasionally they develop encephalitis. Humans can acquire the infection from close contact with infected swine and can develop an encephalitis that may be fatal.

Other swine diseases that occasionally infect humans are swine erysipelas, porcine tuberculosis, and pork tapeworm disease (*cysticercosis*). Swine vesicular disease is primarily confined to pigs but occasionally infects laboratory workers.

Further information can be obtained from the American Association of Swine Veterinarians at www.aasv.org.

Conclusions about Careers with Farm Animals and Horses

Veterinary careers with farm animals and horses can be highly rewarding. They provide exposure to a wide variety of challenging livestock and equine diseases and animal health responsibilities. These careers provide opportunities to become personally involved with hardworking and concerned animal owners who love their animals and often depend upon them for a living. The activities in large animal practice bring veterinarians into contact with varying rural environments, animals, and people.

These activities require round-the-clock availability and application of a wide variety of knowledge, skill, and physical activity that can be exhausting and stressful. When they are pursued in group or corporate practices, the large animal practitioners are provided with time for rest, rehabilitation, and family activities.

Like professional athletes, after 10 to 15 years, the participants in one-man large animal practices may be ready for a change and decide to focus on small animals or move into government, corporate, or academic careers that provide weekend time off and periodic vacations.

In any of these occupations, the years in large animal practice can provide unique experience—both with animals and people. This real-world exposure proves to be invaluable in a variety of other veterinary careers. An excellent book on large animal health is *Keeping Livestock Healthy* by Dr. N. B. Haynes.[6]

The entire veterinary profession, particularly those in academe, is currently struggling to develop methods to convince young people with interests in livestock health to choose careers in veterinary medicine and help address the shortage of livestock veterinarians.

CHAPTER 9

CAREERS IN AVIAN, AQUATIC, LABORATORY, AND ZOO ANIMAL MEDICINE

Introduction

Careers in avian, aquatic, laboratory, and zoo animal medicine comprise unique and rapidly expanding opportunities for veterinarians and veterinary technicians.

These veterinary careers are rarely recognized by young people considering veterinary medicine. Participants in these specialties usually become acquainted with them through lectures heard in veterinary college, through an acquaintance involved in one of these specialties, or through summer employment or a part-time student job.

Avian Medicine

Avian medicine is a growing specialty practiced by keenly focused veterinarians. Most poultry veterinarians are employed by chicken, duck, or turkey producers; universities; diagnostic laboratories; or government agencies.

These veterinarians specialize in the treatment, control, prevention, and diagnosis (often by means of postmortem examination) of poultry diseases. They also conduct disease prevention programs involving vaccinations, nutritional oversight, and environmental stabilization activities. Most avian disease control efforts are exerted at the population level and few efforts are directed at individual animals other than to determine the causes of their illnesses or deaths.

Poultry are affected by a variety of viral, bacterial, and parasitic diseases which require special knowledge and training for their management.

Infectious Diseases of Poultry

The numerous infectious diseases of poultry are mostly caused by viruses and are partially preventable by vaccination. Poultry vaccinations are administered in drinking water or food, as eyedrops, by spraying, or by injection. Diseases for which vaccinations are commonly practiced include avian influenza, Newcastle disease, Marek's disease, infectious anemia, fowlpox, infectious bronchitis, infectious laryngotracheitis, and infectious bursal disease.

Avian influenza infects poultry and wild birds. Many avian influenza virus strains cause mild or unapparent infections, but some pathogenic influenza strains that arise by mutation cause highly fatal outbreaks called fowl plague. A variety of avian influenza vaccines are available.

Newcastle disease is named after the city of Newcastle, England, where it was first studied in detail. It is a globally distributed virus that causes a usually mild respiratory infection and occasional neurologic disorders, which account for its scientific name (avian pneumoencephalitis).

Viscerotropic velogenic Newcastle disease, sometimes called exotic Newcastle disease, results from pathogenic strains which are usually excluded from the United States by import inspections and quarantine measures imposed on imported birds.

When exotic Newcastle disease does gain access to the US, it is eradicated by slaughtering infected flocks, disinfecting the premises, and by controlled restocking. This process was implemented during the 2002–2003 outbreak of exotic Newcastle disease in California.

Marek's disease produces viral-induced tumors in chickens and turkeys. The areas affected include nerves, which often become enlarged, and the intestinal tract and abdominal organs. These lesions sometimes result in death. Marek's disease is usually diagnosed by postmortem examination.

It is partially prevented by vaccination of chicks as they hatch and sometimes the vaccine is inoculated into fertile eggs two to three days before hatching.

Infectious anemia, also called blue wing disease and chicken anemia, is a globally distributed viral infection that occurs mostly in young chickens. It causes loss of appetite, paleness, depression, and sometimes death. Available vaccines are administered by injection or via drinking water to breeding flocks before they begin producing eggs.

Fowlpox is a globally distributed virus infection of chickens and turkeys that causes lumpy scabs on the skin, legs, and sometimes the head. These infections spread slowly by contact but transmission can be accelerated by fighting, mosquito bites, or by contaminated litter.

The causative poxviruses, which differ slightly between chickens and turkeys, can be usually confirmed by the character of the swellings and by microscopic and virologic examination of the lesions.

Fowlpox results in retarded growth and reduced egg production. The secondary bacterial invaders can be reduced by adding antibiotics to the drinking water. Its spread can be slowed by vaccinating chickens and turkeys.

Infectious bronchitis is a rapidly spreading, severe avian respiratory disease characterized by a runny nose, runny eyes, weight loss, and decreased egg production. These signs are present in several other diseases so laboratory tests are required for a definite diagnosis. Several types of infectious bronchitis vaccines are available.

Infectious laryngotracheitis is a severe and often fatal herpesvirus infection of chickens and pheasants. It causes coughing and difficult breathing, loss of appetite, and sometimes tracheal obstruction by mucus. Like many herpesvirus infections, recovered chickens remain carriers and can be the sources of new infections.

The diagnosis of laryngotracheitis can be made by careful observation and is confirmed by postmortem examination and laboratory tests. Infectious laryngotracheitis vaccines are administered via spray, drinking water, or by eyedrops.

Infectious bursal disease, also called Gumboro disease, is a highly contagious, generalized viral infection. The virus is most easily isolated from the fibrous sac lined with a mucus-secreting membrane (bursa) that surrounds the posterior opening into which—in poultry and birds—both the urinary and gastrointestinal tracts empty. Bursal disease is frequently mild and unobserved but can be characterized by severe watery diarrhea, prostration (an abrupt failure of function), and sometimes death. Both newborn chicks and mature hens can be vaccinated against bursal disease.

Pullorum is a highly fatal disease of young chickens and turkeys caused by a bacterium of the genus *Salmonella* (*S. pullorum*) which affects only members of the avian species. Healthy-looking infected birds transmit it through their eggs. Pullorum has been virtually eradicated from commercial poultry flocks by a test-and-slaughter program conducted by the US National Poultry Improvement Program (NPIP).

The test procedure usually uses a veterinarian to collect a drop of blood from under the wing of every bird in a hatchery, deposit it on a glass plate, and add a drop of test antigen. If the hen is infected, the test mixture will precipitate and the donor hen is then caged for transport to the laboratory, where the diagnosis can be verified.

Academic and Industry Careers in Avian Medicine

Most colleges of veterinary medicine have one or more poultry pathologists on the faculty. These specialists present a required course in poultry pathology and diagnose poultry diseases in the college diagnostic laboratories or in postmortem rooms. Most states have an avian disease section in their animal disease diagnostic laboratories.

Many large poultry producers employ a veterinarian, usually an avian disease specialist, who manages their vaccinations and other disease prevention activities, including the health aspects of their nutrition, housing, and management programs.

The American College of Poultry Veterinarians, accessible at www.acvp.info, awards diplomate status to its members based on their formal training and an examination. Further information is also available from the Association of Avian Veterinarians at www.aav.org, from the American Egg Board at www.aeb.org, and from the Mid-Atlantic States Association of Avian Veterinarians at www.MASAAV.org.

Aquatic Animal Medicine

Aquatic animal medicine is a rapidly emerging species specialty. It involves the prevention, diagnosis, treatment, and control of diseases of pet fish and of aquatic animals which are reared commercially for human food. A wide variety of edible fish species including carp, catfish, codfish, halibut, salmon, shrimp, and others are cultivated, grown, and maintained in a variety of settings including tanks, ponds, and net pens in lakes, bays, or oceans. The temperature and sanitation of the environment in which fish are raised is a major factor in their health.

Maintaining profitable health and growth rates for aquatic animals requires adequate nutrition. It also requires cleaning and disinfection of their aquatic habitats and tanks, nets, and all feeding and harvesting equipment. Vaccination programs are being increasingly used in aquaculture programs.

Dietary deficiencies of aquatic animals are being discovered and understood. Because diagnosis of fish diseases is challenging, disease prevention is currently the most effective way of maintaining healthy aquatic populations.

Aquatic mammals such as porpoises and whales are also included in aquatic animal medicine.

The veterinary care of fish used in biomedical research is one phase of laboratory animal medicine. Aquatic animal medicine is expanding and some colleges of veterinary medicine have aquatic animal veterinarians as faculty members who offer elective courses in the area. *The Merck Veterinary Manual*[2] details the veterinary aspects of fish culture.

Fish Diseases

Like other animals and humans, fish are afflicted with bacterial, viral, and fungal infections, and with parasitic infestations. In addition, they are subject to a variety of water contaminants whose toxicities vary for fish species. Many of these conditions are not yet fully understood and can only be diagnosed by postmortem examinations (necropsies). These are most valuable when live or very recently deceased specimens are submitted.

Like most animal species, fish are subject to diseases introduced by the addition of new individuals into established populations. Minimizing introduction of infectious diseases can be accomplished by keeping newly acquired fish under observation in isolation for three to four weeks before adding them to established aquatic populations.

Bacterial infections of fish are common because the water in which they are cultivated can be contaminated with a variety of potential bacterial pathogens which can be fatal for fish stressed by temperature fluctuations, crowding, or competition for food. The specific bacterial causes of fish kills are frequently diagnosed by isolation of bacteria from postmortem specimens. Bacteria are associated with fish diseases named hemorrhagic septicemia, vibriosis, enteric red-mouthed disease, bacterial kidney disease, and many others.

Viral infections of fish are increasingly identified and reported. They are particularly lethal in young fish but can affect fish of all ages. Numerous viruses are being identified and associated with diseases of specific fish species. Aquatic viral infections are usually named by the nature of the disease they cause and by the species of fish they infect.

Some fish diseases are globally distributed, and efforts at their control via limiting importations are under exploration at national and international levels. Some fish infections are listed as reportable diseases by the OIE. Some viral infections of fish appear to be controllable by vaccination, and several vaccines are under development.

Fungal infections are common in cultivated fish and they take a variety of forms. They sometimes occupy the sites of skin injuries, sometimes are secondary invaders to bacterial infections, and less frequently they affect internal organs. Fungi are prominent in aquatic environments, which easily can become contaminated with organic material such as uneaten fish food, unhatched fish eggs, or human, animal, or fish excreta.

Parasitic infestations of fish are numerous and resemble the classifications assigned to both animal and human parasites. They include internal and external protozoan (single-celled) parasites, and wormlike (helminth) parasites which may invade the skin, the gills, or internal organs. Many of these infestations are subclinical and without obvious manifestations.

Some parasitic infestations of pet fish are treated by dipping the fish into disinfectants, or adding chemicals, sulfa drugs, or antibacterial products to the water.

Nutritional disorders of fish are complex and hard to diagnose. Fish require high-protein diets; commercial fish foods meet the needs of some (but not all) farmed fish species. Fish should be fed several times each day, and their eating habits can signal the need for dietary improvement. Most commercial fish foods contain some products of aquatic animal origin.

Several vitamin deficiencies, manifested by retarded growth or other subtle signs, have been documented and most fish diets are supplemented to avoid these hazards.

Water quality is a major challenge to the success of fish farming. Water contaminated with human or animal wastes or decomposed fish food can cause problems.

Veterinarians specializing in aquatic animal medicine continually monitor fish tanks and natural waters housing fish for levels of oxygen, carbon dioxide, salt, chlorine, and ammonia.

These substances can be toxic to each fish species depending on their concentration in the water.

Some common aquatic animal afflictions are preventable by vaccines that are administered by injection or by incorporation into the feed or water. To date, the FDA has approved a limited number of drugs and vaccines for fish, but this process is rapidly advancing.

Aquatic animal medicine is assuming international prominence and the World Organisation for Animal Health (OIE) produces an *International Aquatic Animal Health Code* and the *OIE Manual of Diagnostic Tests and Vaccines for Aquatic Animals*.

For further information, contact the National Aquaculture Association (www.nationalaquaculture.org), the Association of Zoos and Aquariums (www.aza.org), the Society of Aquatic Veterinary Medicine (www.savm.org), or the Association of Reptilian and Amphibian Veterinarians (www.arav.org).

Laboratory Animal Medicine

Laboratory animal medicine is a veterinary specialty that monitors and supervises the use of animals in research on zoonotic and exotic diseases and in a variety of projects that explore basic biological mechanisms. Board-certified specialists in laboratory animal medicine assure that related regulations are followed and that humane and ethical procedures are utilized whenever animals are used for research.

In addition to dogs and cats, a wide variety of experimental animals are used in medical and other research projects. These include baboons, chimpanzees, gerbils, guinea pigs, hamsters, mice, rabbits, rats, and aquatic animals. All of these animals are uniquely suited to differing kinds of testing and investigations of vaccines, drugs and pharmaceuticals, immune pathways, dietary requirements, toxic substances, and antidotes.

The use of animals in research projects is carefully controlled by federal laws, and federally funded research requires humane care and treatment of experimental animals. These requirements demand adequate housing, bedding, feeding, and sanitation for all laboratory animals. The care and use of laboratory animals for research purposes specifically requires supervision by board-certified veterinarians who oversee the laboratory animal facilities and the care, treatment, health, comfort, sanitation, and handling of research animals. Board certification as a laboratory animal veterinarian requires additional training and certification after receipt of the DVM degree.

More information is available from the American College of Laboratory Animal Medicine at www.aclam.org.

Zoo Animal Medicine

Zoo animal medicine is a unique subspecialty that requires special patience, skills, and creativity. Zoo veterinarians are responsible for the health of zoo animals, for the appearance and safety of the animals in confinement, and for their successful reproduction.

These obligations involve the establishment of programs that prevent disease, injuries, and nutritional deficiencies. These programs require balanced diets, appropriate housing, and essential vaccinations. Zoo veterinarians must determine accurate diagnoses and humanely administer appropriate treatments when animals are sick or injured.

Zoo Animal Disease Prevention Programs

Disease prevention programs for zoo animals are complex and challenging undertakings. Although wild animals living in captivity in zoos suffer from diseases and parasites that are similar—and often identical—to those experienced by domestic species, the treatment, prevention, and control of these conditions in zoos provides exceptional challenges.

It is essential to quarantine newly acquired individuals or groups of animals, birds, or reptiles in cleaned and disinfected isolation facilities prior to placing them in their permanent locations in a zoo. During the quarantine period, they must be observed daily for any evidence of infectious diseases or parasites and vaccinated against diseases specific to their species. Once established in their environmentally compatible quarters, they are observed regularly to assure that rivalries don't erupt into combat. They must also be observed carefully for signs of malnutrition or disease.

Zoo Animal Examinations and Disease Diagnosis

Disease diagnosis among caged animals in zoos requires careful examination of their eating and sleeping habits and their social interactions with their companions in the yards or pens.

Upon any sign of disease or upset, the suspicious animals require containment and examination by the veterinarian, samples need to be collected for diagnostic purposes, and the animal must be isolated if infectious diseases are suspected.

Treatment of Diseases and Injuries of Zoo Animals

The treatment of diseases and injuries of zoo animals requires patience, tact, caution, and strict attention to the safety of both the caregivers and the patients. The administration of medications requires careful restraint to avoid injuries and cautious attention to dosages. Most zoos have creative techniques, devices, and facilities for trapping and restraining animals for diagnostic examinations, for collection of appropriate samples, and for administration of medications.

Repair of fractures, bleeding wounds, and other injuries often requires general anesthesia that must be carefully administered in doses estimated to be effective and safe.

The Merck Veterinary Manual[2] provides an excellent description of the veterinary aspects of zoo animal medicine, and the American College of Zoological Medicine (www.aczm.org) can provide further information.

Summary of Careers in Avian, Aquatic, Laboratory, and Zoo Animal Medicine

Careers in avian, aquatic, laboratory, and zoo animal medicine can be exciting, challenging, and filled with variety. These careers offer an ever-changing professional environment.

Experts in these areas can readily find employment in academe, government, and industry. The unique challenges of these specialties offer opportunities to bind with like-minded colleagues at association meetings and provide frequent invitations to lecture at colleges and meetings.

CHAPTER 10
DISCIPLINE-SPECIFIC VETERINARY SPECIALTIES

Introduction

In veterinary medicine, discipline-specific specialties are carried out by private practitioners and by academic, corporate, or governmental employees. Discipline specialties can involve body systems such as the heart (cardiology) and the eyes (ophthalmology), and causes of diseases such as poisons (toxicology) or parasites (parasitology). There are also curative specialties such as surgery and pharmacology. Specialists in disease prevention work in disciplines such as veterinary public health and epidemiology. In addition, there are other combinations that include several areas.

Veterinary discipline specialists serve herds, flocks, or individual animals with diagnostic or treatment procedures. In academic environments (colleges of veterinary medicine or departments of veterinary science, for example), they lecture to students, perform diagnostic tests and procedures, and provide treatments for diseases and injuries.

Most discipline-specific specialties involve the basic subjects studied in veterinary colleges. Disciplinary specialists at universities are usually expected to teach and conduct research projects or exploratory procedures, which are fully completed only when published in professional journals or described in written summaries of talks at scientific meetings.

There are textbooks written by experts in most fields that explain discipline-specific specialties. These books are usually required reading for students taking the related courses and must be updated frequently to accommodate new information.

The following list of discipline-specific veterinary specialties resembles the list of required courses taught in veterinary colleges.

Anatomy

Veterinary anatomy addresses the structural details of animals and their parts. Anatomy is learned by separating and studying animal parts to ascertain their location and their positional and functional relationships with other bodily structures.

Anatomy classes have some lectures, but they mostly involve laboratories in which students dissect embalmed cadavers or manipulate plastic replicas of anatomic structures.

The dissections and manipulations are guided by professors and laboratory assistants and are illustrated and detailed in textbooks or dissection guides which provide stepwise instructions.

Veterinary anatomy is considered a basic science and is taught in the first and second semesters at most veterinary colleges. All veterinary colleges have one or more professors of anatomy who are largely occupied with teaching, but they are also expected to publish articles in scientific journals.

Anatomic Pathology

Anatomic pathology is the study of changes in body tissues and organs as determined by the naked eye during surgery, by clinical examination, or by postmortem examinations.

Almost all colleges of veterinary medicine have a postmortem room for examination of animals that succumb in the college clinics and for deceased animals submitted by practitioners or delivered by animal owners.

Postmortem rooms are staffed by experienced veterinary pathologists who render an initial diagnosis based on gross anatomic findings. These diagnoses are subject to substantiation by laboratory tests and by microscopic (histopathologic) examination of tissue specimens.

Nonacademic facilities that use laboratory animals for research also have postmortem facilities and veterinarians to conduct necropsies. More information about pathology is available from the American College of Veterinary Pathologists at their website, www.acvp.org.

Animal Behavior

Veterinarians specializing in animal behavior study the causes, diagnosis, treatment, prevention, and control of undesirable mental, physical, emotional, or attitudinal problems exhibited by animals. These include unwillingness to be housebroken, aggressive activities, and unwillingness to be trained.

The discipline of animal behavior has blossomed in the past 50 years, and canine, feline, and equine behaviorists are kept busy examining pets, consulting with their owners, and lecturing on the subject to students and audiences of animal lovers or veterinarians. Most veterinary colleges offer elective or required courses in animal behavior and many veterinary meetings present programs on the subject.

The American College of Veterinary Behaviorists at www.dacvb.org certifies animal behavior diplomates based on an examination.

Anesthesiology

Veterinary anesthesiologists specialize in rendering animals insensitive to pain so that potentially painful surgery or other procedures can be effectively performed. Anesthesiologists must have clinical and research experience and be familiar with anesthetic agents, the procedures for their administration, their safe dosages, their toxic effects, and their antidotes.

Anesthesiologists are experts in supporting the life of patients under anesthesia and the management of unconscious patients. Veterinary anesthesiologists with adequate clinical or research experience are board certified by the American College of Veterinary Anesthesiologists (www.acva.org).

Cardiology

Veterinary cardiologists work mostly with dogs and cats and occasionally with horses and other species. They are experts in diagnosing and treating heart disorders and using stethoscopes and equipment such as ultrasound devices, fluoroscopy, computer tomography (CT), and magnetic resonance imaging (MRI).

They also perform heart surgery and monitor the heart actions of animals under anesthesia. Most veterinary colleges have cardiologists who teach and perform clinical services.

Clinical Pathology

Veterinary clinical pathology is the diagnosis of animal disease by means of laboratory tests. Each veterinary college has a clinical pathology laboratory staffed by board-certified clinical pathologists and veterinary technicians. Clinical pathologists run diagnostic tests on blood, urine, feces, and skin scrapings of all species.

After academic clinicians examine patients, unless the diagnosis is obvious, they develop a list (called a differential diagnosis) of possible causes of an animal's problem. Then they collect appropriate samples and submit them to the clinical pathology laboratory for analysis.

The clinical pathologists, who are experts at running and interpreting tests, evaluate the test results, rule out unlikely diagnoses, and offer opinions or specifics about the cause of the problem.

More information is available from the American Society for Veterinary Clinical Pathology (www.asvcp.org).

Dermatology

Dermatology is the study of the structure, function, and diseases of the skin. Veterinary dermatologists address skin problems of all species of animals but most of their activity involves pets. Skin disorders can be caused by bacteria, fungi, parasites, tumors, allergies, or hormonal disorders. Skin diseases frequently persist through long periods of treatment, so veterinary dermatologists become very familiar with their patients and their owners.

The American Academy of Veterinary Dermatology (www.aavd.org) provides further information. Board certification conferred by the American College of Veterinary Dermatology (www.acvd.org) is based on an examination plus a one-year internship and two or more years' experience in the diagnosis and treatment of skin disorders.

Emergency Medicine and Critical Care

The specialty of emergency medicine and critical care is an important component of companion animal medicine. The number of emergency clinics for dog, cat, and horse patients is expanding rapidly so that emergency veterinary services are available at night and on weekends and holidays.

Some emergency clinics are run by one or more private practitioners and others are run by groups of neighboring practitioners who take turns manning the operation when their own hospital is closed.

The American College of Veterinary Emergency and Critical Care at www.acvecc.org and the Veterinary Emergency and Critical Care Society at www.veccs.org have further information.

Epidemiology

Epidemiology is the study of the distribution of diseases in populations. Epidemiologists estimate the incidence and prevalence of diseases and compare data to determine changes that improve the health of animal populations or problems that may require regulatory intervention.

Epidemiologic studies of the incidence (new cases per unit of population in given time intervals) and prevalence (the number of existing cases per unit of population at a given time) are used to identify population-based disease issues. Thus, epidemiologists work with numbers to devise disease control and prevention strategies.

Veterinary epidemiologists also investigate unusual outbreaks of diseases in animal populations. They interview owners about sick animals, the introduction of new animals, possible changes in diet or management routines, recent construction, storm damage, or changes in fertilization and insecticide application procedures.

During investigations, they examine the premises for waste disposal sites which may be accessible to animals and for fencing problems. They also check the highway boundaries for discarded trash. After completing this process, they examine healthy animals and finally the sick ones to establish diagnostic possibilities and develop a differential diagnosis which can be confirmed by laboratory tests or necropsy.

Further information about veterinary epidemiology is available from the American College of Veterinary Preventative Medicine at www.acvpm.org, the American Epidemiology Society at www.hartz.com, and the Association for Veterinary Epidemiology and Preventative Medicine which can be contacted on the Internet at www.cvm.uiuc.edu/avepm.

Histology and Histopathology

Histology is the study of the microscopic structure of normal tissues. It provides essential background for histopathology, the microscopic examination and study of abnormal or diseased tissues. Histopathologists need a thorough understanding of the appearance of normal tissues in order to recognize abnormalities.

A course in histology is a prerequisite for admission to some veterinary colleges and is part of the first-year curriculum of others. Normal histology is constantly reviewed during diagnostic examination of animal tissues. The examination of organ and tissue specimens for diagnostic purposes helps determine the most appropriate therapeutic procedures and the potential outcome of treatments.

Internal Medicine

Internal veterinary medicine is the study of physiologic and pathologic characteristics of the internal organs and the diagnosis and treatment of conditions which are not apparent by the external examination of affected animals.

Internal medicine is practiced in many veterinary procedures. The American College of Veterinary Internal Medicine (www.acvim.org) offers board certification in subspecialties of cardiology, neurology, oncology, and large animal and small animal internal medicine.

Microbiology and Immunology

Microbiology is the study of organisms invisible to the naked eye. Veterinary microbiologists teach the characteristics, life cycles, and methods for detection of bacterial, viral, fungal, and other microscopic agents that cause disease. The subsets of veterinary microbiology are bacteriology, virology, immunology, serology, and microscopic parasitology.

Bacterial infections and diseases are usually transmitted by contaminated soil, feces, urine, or other bodily discharges. Viral diseases are usually transmitted by bodily fluids or insect bites.

In the early years of veterinary medical curriculums, courses are presented in bacteriology, virology, and microscopic parasitology. Further information is available from the website of the American College of Veterinary Microbiologists, which can be reached at www.vetmed.iastate.edu/acvm.

Immunology, which is related to microbiology as a subset, is the study of the body's reaction to foreign antigens (substances that stimulate immune responses). Antibodies are responses to foreign antigens and can be detected in body fluids. Blood tests for infections analyze the clear portion of the blood (serum) for antibodies, with a variety of laboratory procedures collectively called serology.

Nephrology

Nephrology is the study of the anatomy, physiology, and pathology of the kidneys. Veterinarians who specialize in the diagnosis and treatment of kidney diseases and tumors usually also have expertise in the normal and abnormal functioning of the entire urinary system.

Thus, nephrologists sometimes deal with disorders of the urethra and bladder as well as the kidneys. They rely on urinalysis as a diagnostic tool. The Society of Veterinary Nephrology and Urology at www.umn.edu can provide further information.

Neurology

Neurology deals with diseases of the nervous system including the brain, spinal cord, and nerves. These disorders can result from bacteria, viral, or fungal infections; parasitic invasions; poisonings; trauma; congenital disorders; or tumors. It is often challenging to identify nervous disorders of animals, to diagnose them, and to determine their cause. Neurological infections include most animal encephalitides and rabies.

Rabies can affect most animal species, is usually fatal, and is a challenging disease to diagnose in its early stages. Most mosquito-borne viral animal encephalitides can infect humans, and some can be fatal for people.

Nutrition

Each animal species has specific nutritional requirements for health, survival, growth, and reproductive efficiency. Nutritional stages include ingestion, digestion, absorption, and utilization. Sound nutrition is essential for all animal species, and nutritional deficiencies or excesses can cause health problems.

Veterinary nutritionists monitor intake and check blood levels of water, proteins, carbohydrates, vitamins, and minerals. Livestock nutrition is a major component of the educational, research, and public information activities of every college of agriculture and school of veterinary medicine. American colleges of veterinary medicine usually have cooperative livestock nutritional teaching and research programs with agricultural colleges.

Further information can be found at the American Academy of Veterinary Nutrition at www.aavn.org and the American College of Veterinary Nutrition at www.acvn.org.

Ophthalmology

Veterinary ophthalmologists study the anatomy, physiology, functions, and pathology of the eyes of animals. They diagnose and treat ocular disorders using a variety of medical and surgical techniques.

Ophthalmologists at colleges of veterinary medicine work closely with small animal and large animal clinicians and with students. They present lectures on eye disorders.

Some ophthalmologists have private practices in which they accept referrals of animals with eye problems from small animal and general practitioners. They are experts in the diagnosis and treatment of eye disorders and the appropriate corrective surgery.

Further information is available from the American College of Veterinary Ophthalmologists at www.acvo.org and the American Society of Veterinary Ophthalmology at www.asvo.org.

Parasitology

Parasites are organisms that live on or in host animals and obtain nourishment from them. There are internal and external parasites and facultative and obligatory parasites. Facultative parasites can survive independent of their host animal, while obligatory parasites require host animals for survival.

Some parasites are transmitted by biting insects, and others are acquired by ingestion of parasite eggs in fecal-contaminated grass or other foodstuffs.

Skin parasites can be diagnosed by external examination, gastrointestinal parasites are detected by microscopic exam of feces, and blood parasites are identified by microscopic examination of blood samples.

Veterinary colleges have parasitology professors who teach required courses on the subject. More information can be obtained from the American Association of Veterinary Parasitologists (www.aavp.org).

Pathology

Pathology is the study of the characteristics, causes, and effects of disease on body structure and function. Pathologists teach required courses in veterinary colleges and diagnose diseases in specially equipped postmortem rooms in universities, regional veterinary diagnostic laboratories, and research institutions.

Pathologists assess grossly visible lesions and microscopic (histopathologic) abnormalities or changes in body tissues. Lesions are subdivided into gross or microscopic, benign or malignant, and primary or secondary.

Further information is available from the American College of Veterinary Pathologists at www.acvp.org.

Pharmacology

Pharmacology is the study of the nomenclature, preparation, properties, uses, actions, and antidotes of drugs and biological products used in the treatment and prevention of diseases. Most colleges of veterinary medicine have required courses in pharmacology early in their curriculums. Experienced veterinary pharmacologists are often hired by firms that develop and market animal drugs. More information is available from the American Academy of Veterinary Pharmacology and Therapeutics at www.aavpt.org.

Preventive Medicine

Preventive veterinary medicine is a branch of health care concerned with implementing—on a population basis—the maintenance of herd and flock health through disease prevention, nutritional management, and environmental measures.

Preventive medicine specialists seek methods of preventing infectious and noninfectious diseases. These measures include security, vaccination, premises and personnel disinfection, nutritional and environmental adjustments, and sanitary measures for people working with animals. This sometimes requires showering by all people entering or leaving animal quarters.

These specialists limit the spread of infectious agents by vaccination, appropriate sanitary measures, careful monitoring to increase likelihood of early recognition and diagnosis of diseases, and by eliminating disease-supporting activities. Consult the

Association for Veterinary Epidemiology and Preventive Medicine at www.cvm.uiuc.edu/avepm.

Public Health

Veterinary public health is the branch of veterinary medicine that deals with the role of animals and animal products in human health. Veterinarians play key roles in human health agencies in every state and at the national level. Zoonotic diseases—including bacterial, fungal, parasitic, and viral afflictions—are animal diseases that can be transmitted to humans. Some of these, such as brucellosis, tuberculosis, and rabies, result from direct contact with animals. Others—like trichinosis and some food poisonings—are transmitted by improperly cooked foods of animal origin. Still others, like the viral encephalitides, are transmitted from animals to people via insects. Some other zoonoses, like tetanus, result from direct or indirect human contact with animal wastes.

The Merck Veterinary Manual[2] lists over 150 diseases that are transmitted from animals to humans. These include 32 bacterial diseases, 12 rickettsial diseases, 13 fungal diseases, 12 protozoal diseases, 36 other parasitic diseases, 6 arthropod-borne diseases, 51 viral diseases, and 1 prion-induced disease. Many of these can also be spread by human-to-human transmission.

Information can be obtained from the National Association of State Public Health Veterinarians at www.nasphv.org and from the Office of the Chief Veterinarian of the US Public Health Service at www.usphs.gov.html/vet.cpo.html.

Radiology and Radiation Oncology

Radiology is the use of X-rays in the diagnosis and treatment of diseases. Every college of veterinary medicine has one or more radiologists on their faculty. They teach radiology courses and perform diagnostic and therapeutic procedures which utilize radiology. Veterinary radiologists mostly use radiological techniques for visualization of bodily structures for diagnostic purposes. In addition, some practice radiation oncology for the treatment of cancer.

Further information is available from the American College of Veterinary Radiology at www.acvr.org.

Surgery

Surgery is the use of operative procedures to correct tissue damage resulting from trauma or medical conditions. There are also many routine veterinary surgeries such as spaying of females and neutering of males, and dehorning of calves and goats. Some surgical procedures (tail docking and ear cropping of dogs) are controversial. Each animal species has a variety of routine and emergency medical conditions that require surgical treatment.

Each college of veterinary medicine has several small animal surgeons who serve the small animal clinic and large animal surgeons who operate on sheep, goats, cattle, and horses, both on farms and in the teaching hospital. They usually have students and interns serving as assistants. They also deliver lectures and preside over surgical teaching laboratories which sometimes use artificial animals as teaching models.

More information on veterinary surgery is available from the American College of Veterinary Surgeons at www.acvs.org.

Theriogenology (Animal Reproduction)

Theriogenology means animal reproduction. There are both large animal theriogenologists and small animal theriogenologists. They both work to improve reproductive efficiency of animals. A major part of their efforts involves determining the presence of pregnancy. In cattle and horses, this is accomplished by palpating the uterus, which is accessible by entering the rectum with a gloved hand and arm. In smaller species, this procedure is not possible and other approaches, such as gentle manual palpation of the abdomen, and radiology, are used.

Theriogenologists develop expertise in identifying the causes of animal infertility and in diagnosing diseases of the female and male reproductive organs.

More information can be obtained from the American College of Theriogenologists (www.theriogenology.org), the American Embryo Transfer Association (www.aeta.org), and the Society for Theriogenology at www.therio.org.

Toxicology

Veterinary toxicologists usually work in diagnostic or research laboratories where they analyze body tissues, blood, urine, feces, and environmental specimens for the presence of potentially poisonous substances. In academe, toxicologists present toxicology courses, perform diagnostic tests, and conduct research.

Veterinary toxicologists have special training in the diagnosis and treatment of animal poisonings. They have understanding, gained through knowledge and experience, of the structure, functions, and effects on bodily functions of natural and manmade, organic and inorganic, substances and plant toxins and their dose-response relationships in each animal species.

Board certification in veterinary toxicology requires the DVM degree plus an advanced degree and publications in the field. Further information is available from the American Board of Veterinary Toxicology at www.abvt.org.

Veterinary Medical Extension

Veterinary extension agents, partly supported by state and federal extension programs, deliver information to pet and livestock owners, farmers, and veterinarians. They consult with clients who have problems, lecture at meetings, and write timely news items of public interest on animal health issues.

When hired by colleges of veterinary medicine at universities, veterinary extension agents must demonstrate field experience and be excellent speakers and credible writers.

Extension agents keep abreast of emerging issues in their field and advise the public of necessary disease prevention measures. They are familiar with state and federal regulations that involve animals and animal products, and they understand the animal diseases which are communicable to humans.

The American Association of Extension Veterinarians meets annually, usually in association with the AVMA meeting, to keep their membership apprised of current issues.

Summary of Disciplinary Specialties

Most disciplinary specialties require formal advanced training acquired through internships, residencies, board certifications, or graduate programs. Veterinarians become acquainted with many disciplinary specialists whom they encounter as teachers, regulators, corporate employees, or representatives of various veterinary organizations, in jobs where they focus intensely on an area of their special interest.

Usually the narrow focus of their specialty permits a thorough and detailed knowledge of an area about which most veterinarians have more general knowledge. Thus they acquire reputations as experts, are called upon as consultants, and are invited to speak at meetings. Their reputations are greatly enhanced if they write a book about their chosen subject.

CHAPTER 11

VETERINARY AND ANIMAL HEALTH ORGANIZATIONS

Introduction

There are many local, state, national, and global veterinary organizations that focus on individual scientific disciplines, practice types, animal species, or animal health policies. These correspond to some extent to the clubs that students join in college and reflect interests that veterinarians acquire over the years.

There are too many veterinary associations, academies, boards, institutes, and societies for any veterinarian to belong to them all. However, most veterinarians participate actively in one or more veterinary organizations or college groups to stay current in their field and maintain contact with colleagues.

Potential applicants to colleges of veterinary medicine will be interested in the vast array of veterinary and animal health organizations in which the members of the profession participate. Most of the organizations described below hold annual meetings. They are but a small sample of the many groups that serve the interests of veterinarians.

The American Veterinary Medical Association

The American Veterinary Medical Association (AVMA) is the major all-purpose US veterinary organization. Most of the estimated 85,000 plus veterinarians in the United States are AVMA members.

The AVMA has suborganizations that focus on animal species and disciplinary specialties. It works to gain public support for issues involving: the care, health, and comfort of pets, poultry, and livestock; the prevention and control of human diseases acquired from animals; and the improvement of the health and safety of foods of animal origin. The AVMA meets annually at various locations throughout the United States. The meetings include committee, council, and task force meetings in many areas and programs on many veterinary topics.

The AVMA House of Delegates has representatives from every state. They constantly amend the bylaws and adjust AVMA positions on national and international issues that affect the profession.

The Auxiliary to the AVMA offers networking opportunities for veterinary families, provides student loans and scholarships, and promotes animal welfare. See www.avmaaux.org.

AVMA Publications

The AVMA produces three publications. These are the *Journal of the American Veterinary Medical Association* (*JAVMA*), the *American Journal of Veterinary Research* (*AJVR*), and the *AVMA Membership Directory & Resource Manual*.[7]

The *JAVMA* is published on the first and fifteenth day of each month and is mailed to all AVMA members. It contains news of the profession, practice-oriented scientific reports, meeting announcements, employment opportunities, obituaries, and commentary on legislation related to animals.

The *JAVMA* has an editorial board and its scientific articles are considered refereed papers.

The *AJVR* is a prestigious refereed monthly research publication. It is available to members in lieu of receiving the *JAVMA* or for an additional charge. The *AJVR* contains detailed research reports on issues involving animals and the veterinary profession.

The *AVMA Membership Directory & Resource Manual*[7] is a comprehensive volume on the US veterinary profession. It lists the names and addresses of veterinarians both alphabetically and by state and hometown. It also provides the names of the members of specialty groups, and the name, address, and leadership of every US and Canadian college of veterinary medicine. In addition, the directory lists the names and e-mail addresses of all state and local veterinary organizations, societies, and specialty boards.

Prospective veterinary students may wish to ask a veterinarian for permission to peruse these AVMA publications.

The AVMA Councils

The AVMA has seven elected councils that oversee various areas of veterinary medicine. They include: the Council on Biological and Therapeutic Agents, the Council on Communications, the

Council on Education, the Judicial Council, the Council on Public Health and Regulatory Medicine, the Council on Research, and the Council on Veterinary Service. Each council recommends positions and actions that will support the best interests of animal health, the veterinary profession, and the public at large.

The AVMA Council on Education (COE) has about 20 elected members representing various phases of the profession. It establishes and updates the standards by which colleges of veterinary medicine are accredited.

The COE regularly evaluates each college regarding "Standards of an Accredited College of Veterinary Medicine." These standards include: organization, finances, physical facilities and equipment, clinical resources, library resources, students, admissions, faculty, curriculum, research programs, and outcomes assessment. The COE evaluates these standards by examining a required self-study report produced by each college and by site visits.

The COE assigns a classification of Provisional Accreditation, Full Accreditation, Limited Accreditation, Terminal Accreditation, or Reasonable Assurance to each college.

The AVMA Mission

The AVMA establishes standards for the profession through participatory policy development and enforces these standards in a variety of ways.

The AVMA headquarters in Schaumburg, Illinois, houses most full-time AVMA staffers and serves as one site for meetings of elected officers, councils, and committees. However, some full-time staffers are housed at the AVMA Government Relations Office in Washington, DC.

State Veterinary Medical Associations

Every US state has a veterinary medical association that addresses the state's animal health and animal-related human health needs. State veterinary societies provide up-to-date information on emerging diseases and issues. They also exert political pressure in areas of veterinary concern.

State associations have annual meetings that provide updates on statewide issues involving the profession and on changing regulations that affect animals and animal health. They also present programs that deal with animal diseases. State veterinary meetings permit practitioners to discuss ideas with colleagues in practice, government, and industry.

Some state veterinary associations also have infrastructural and disciplinary functions. They influence and sometimes actually manage state licensing procedures, and investigate malpractice claims. They offer advice to government officials about the design and execution of animal health regulations and about requirements for moving animals across state lines.

Within states, there are county or multicounty associations that address similar issues on a local basis and provide social interactions among veterinarians and their families. These organizations serve to create cooperation among practitioners. They also contact state legislators on issues of veterinary significance.

The Association of American Veterinary Medical Colleges (AAVMC)

The Association of American Veterinary Medical Colleges (AAVMC) is an organization that comprises the leadership and the faculty of all 32 US and Canadian colleges of veterinary medicine.

Its members also include nine departments of veterinary science in colleges of agriculture, seven departments of comparative medicine in medical schools, and six international colleges of veterinary medicine.

The AAVMC works with government agencies, veterinary medical associations, and animal and human health organizations to strengthen veterinary education in North America and throughout the world.

The AAVMC manages a centralized application program for US and Canadian veterinary colleges and some international institutions. It is called the Veterinary Medical College Application Service (VMCAS) and is described in chapter four.

The AAVMC Diversity Program

The AAVMC works to increase diversity in the profession by increasing the variety of students in veterinary colleges. This is an effort to overcome the profession's longstanding student imbalances regarding race, color, gender, and national backgrounds. Once dominated by white males, veterinary college students are now mostly female.

The AAVMC is trying to achieve a student body that approximates the distribution of people in the US population. This effort has programs for administrators, admission committees, and veterinary organizations in an effort to encourage diversity. The program establishes diversity committees in individual colleges and stimulates veterinary associations to focus on diversity.

Efforts to stimulate interest in veterinary medicine among minorities are also directed at elementary, middle school, junior high, and senior high school students.

Global Initiatives in Veterinary Education

The AAVMC has a program called Global Initiatives in Veterinary Education (GIVE) that encourages long-term, meaningful partnerships between North American veterinary schools and companion colleges in developing countries.

Under the aegis of GIVE, AAVMC member colleges and cooperating organizations supply books, journals, instruments, equipment, and curricular materials, and encourage exchanges of faculty and students.

Other AAVMC Programs

The AAVMC grants a number of awards and prizes that stimulate changes in college programs and curriculums. They encourage curriculum improvements, increased teaching effectiveness, and distribution of information about careers in veterinary medicine.

At the AAVMC annual meetings held near their home office in Washington, DC, they present programs that update attendees on current educational issues. They also lobby legislators for improved funding for veterinary medical education and for college facilities.

The AAVMC Long-Range Plan for Veterinary Education

During 2006 and 2007, the AAVMC undertook a foresight project called "Envisioning the Future of Veterinary Education"[8] to develop long-range directions for US and Canadian colleges of veterinary medicine over the next 10 to 25 years.

Over 95 individuals from a variety of animal health occupations and academic and practice specialties discussed the challenges facing veterinary education. Some of these issues are discussed in chapter twelve.

The participants concluded: that there are inadequate numbers of veterinarians to address the changing needs of society in food animal medicine, biomedical research, public health, and companion animal medicine; that colleges of veterinary medicine must address these needs; that the profession must convince society of its vital role in changing times; and that veterinary colleges must collectively address these needs by having each college offer specialized training available to students from the rest of North America.

Meeting these needs will probably require increased class sizes, accreditation of veterinary colleges which do not offer clinical training in all fields, and adjustment of veterinary licensing flexibility. The panel recommended that the AAVMC take the leadership in meeting these challenges. The AAVMC has responded by establishing a task force to address them.

The US Animal Health Association (USAHA)

The United States Animal Health Association (USAHA) was established in 1897 under a different name. It is a collection of organizations and individuals dedicated to improving and stabilizing the health of US and global livestock populations.

It has about 1,400 members representing all aspects of animal and human health. Most of its members belong to other related organizations and many are official representatives of government agencies, corporations, or specialty groups.

The annual USAHA meetings are held in conjunction with the American Association of Veterinary Laboratory Diagnosticians. At these joint meetings, committees discuss a wide variety of issues and present recommendations and resolutions that encourage state and federal agencies to undertake programs to support animal and human health. USAHA lobbies state and federal governments.

The National Institute for Animal Agriculture (NIAA)

The National Institute for Animal Agriculture (NIAA) was initiated in 1916 as the Sanitary Committee of the Chicago Livestock Exchange. It has gone by several names including the National Livestock Loss Prevention Board and the Livestock

Conservation Institute. In 2000 it became the NIAA. For almost a century it has focused on issues concerning livestock production, marketing, and health.

Its membership is a diverse mixture of livestock producers, regulators, scientists, and veterinarians representing private, organizational, corporate, governmental, and academic practice.

NIAA provides a forum for building consensus-based solutions to the challenges of animal agriculture. They provide educational programs and serve to connect professionals in the field of animal agriculture. See www.animalagriculture.org for further NIAA information.

The National Association of State Universities and Land Grant Colleges (NASULGC)

The National Association of State Universities and Land Grant Colleges, founded in 1887, is the nation's oldest higher education organization. Its membership includes the leadership of US educational institutions that receive federal funding.

Land-grant universities were established by the Morrill Act of 1862 and the Hatch Act of 1887 which provided land for agricultural experiment stations at state universities. By 1890, federal programs had donated over 11 million acres of land for public universities.

NASULGC holds annual meetings and special subject conferences that support teaching excellence, student aid, and academic freedom. They encourage study abroad, cooperation between US and foreign universities, research and development activities, and extension programs.

NASULGC is the major communication organization between public universities and US state and federal governments. It works to keep state and federal legislators apprised of the status, public value, progress, and needs of the nation's higher education system.

The Humane Society of the United States (HSUS)

The Humane Society of the United States (HSUS) and its members pursue sustainable humane conditions for all animals, including pets, livestock, and wildlife, by working to reduce animal suffering, by supporting local humane societies, and by undertaking legislative actions that ensure their goals.

The HSUS has teamed with the AVMA and other veterinary organizations to improve humane treatment for animals of all species. They can be contacted at www.hsus.org.

The Council for Agricultural Science and Technology (CAST)

The Council for Agricultural Science and Technology (CAST) is an organization of scientific societies and individuals. It prepares task force reports and issue papers. CAST documents contain scientifically accurate information in formats understandable to the general public.

These documents cover issues such as vaccines for avian influenza, resource preservation, environmental toxins, water quality, agricultural policies, and more. They are distributed to the scientific community, to legislators, to policymakers, and to the media with the intent to educate. CAST can be contacted at www.cast-science.org.

The National Association of Federal Veterinarians (NAFV)

The National Association of Federal Veterinarians (NAFV) serves as the organized voice of about 2,400 federally employed veterinarians. Its members work for the Food and Drug Administration, the Department of Agriculture, the US military, and other government agencies.

The NAFV has elected officers and an executive vice president and a staff assistant in its Washington, DC, office. It meets in conjunction with the annual meetings of the AVMA and the USAHA. Further information is available at www.nafv.org.

A similar organization that represents most state-employed veterinarians is called the National Association of State Public Health Veterinarians. It is accessible at www.nasphv.org.

The North American Veterinary Conference (NAVC)

The North American Veterinary Conference (NAVC) is an organization that provides continuing education and family-oriented vacation activities.

This mission is accomplished with an annual Florida-based January conference for practitioners, students, receptionists, practice managers, and technologists who work to address the needs of animals. NAVC provides proceedings books from the sections on small and large animal medicine and veterinary technology. There are other regionally based annual veterinary meetings, including the Western Veterinary Conference, which is held in Las Vegas, Nevada, in February.

The National Academies of Practice (NAP)

The National Academies of Practice (NAP) is a coalition of dentists, nurses, osteopaths, pharmacists, physicians, and veterinarians. It is a broad-based interdisciplinary organization that works to impact public policy and programs. It strives to assure that health services are available to everyone. It achieves these goals through lobbying and public policy statements assembled by panels of health care workers and experts.

The Pan American Health Organization (PAHO)

The Pan American Health Organization (PAHO) promotes human health throughout the Americas. It addresses zoonotic diseases and has programs aimed at putting good health within the reach of all people, including neglected, vulnerable, marginalized, and excluded populations.

Many PAHO efforts facilitate dialog among educators and decision makers to ensure effective distribution of health resources throughout the Americas. For further information, contact PAHO at www.paho.org.

The Animal Health Institute (AHI)

The Animal Health Institute (AHI) is an organization of research companies and manufacturers of pharmaceuticals, biological products, vaccines, insecticides, and pesticides that improve the health and well-being of animals. By so doing, these products also protect human health.

AHI members represent corporations and government agencies dedicated to creating a stable and safe society by encouraging scientifically sound regulatory environments that assure the safety and efficacy of animal health products. For further information, go to www.ahi.org.

The National Association of Veterinary Technicians in America (NAVTA)

The National Association of Veterinary Technicians in America (NAVTA) represents veterinary technicians and technologists that provide technical support to veterinarians and biomedical research personnel. They also work to assure high standards of animal care in veterinary clinics.

NAVTA provides information at meetings and publishes a professional journal to update its members, who handle patient care and laboratory procedures under the supervision of veterinarians.

In addition to working with and supporting practitioners, veterinary technicians and technologists work in academe, humane societies, diagnostic laboratories, industry, and with the military. Some help design and implement research animal facilities. More information on how veterinary technologists help serve the public and the profession is available at www.navta.net.

The Office International des Épizooties (OIE)

The Office International des Épizooties is now called the **World Organisation for Animal Health**, but it retains its original initialization (OIE).

The OIE is the world's oldest international veterinary organization. It was formed in 1924, is headquartered in Paris, France, and has about 160 member countries. Its goals are to insure transparency in global animal health issues, develop and maintain a worldwide animal disease reporting network, and to facilitate world trade by minimizing the risk of spreading livestock diseases.

The OIE meets each year at its Paris headquarters. At this meeting, the official delegates and the alternate delegates sit in assigned seats in the auditorium and the rest of each country's delegation sits in back. Speakers talk into microphones and all listeners have headsets with language selectors to choose between Arabic, English, French, German, and Russian translations. The delegation from the US involves the leadership of major animal health organizations.

The annual OIE meeting is attended by Chief Veterinary Officers (CVOs) and accompanying delegations from member countries. Each country's CVO is the sole voting delegate and each country has one vote despite the country's size or population. National delegations include national and subnational veterinary officials and representatives of some nongovernmental organizations (NGOs).

The OIE is the international standards–setting organization for livestock health. It maintains an animal disease reporting system; prepares criteria for disease-free status of countries; and recommends sanitary measures such as testing, quarantine, and health certification procedures for safe international trade in animals and livestock products.

The US delegation usually includes representatives from the USAHA, the AVMA, the academic and diagnostic communities, the United States Department of Agriculture, and state veterinary officers. The annual OIE meeting provides opportunities for veterinary officials from around the world to meet formally and network informally.

The OIE uses regionally balanced expert working groups to develop draft standards which are circulated for comment prior to adoption. Comments are accepted only from delegates. Most delegates involve their scientific, regulatory, agricultural, and veterinary communities in the process. This communication strengthens the delegate's effectiveness. Despite occasional efforts to politicize them, OIE standards are usually based on sound science.

OIE standards are adopted, usually by consensus, by the General Assembly at annual meetings. If there is a call for a vote, there is one vote per country. The OIE international standards are published and regularly updated in the *OIE Codes*.

The OIE International Animal Health Code

The OIE publishes an *International Terrestrial Animal Health Code. The Code* describes livestock diseases and recommended testing, vaccination, health certification, and quarantine measures needed for safe international movement of livestock, poultry, semen, and related commodities.

They also publish a similar *Aquatic Animal Health Code* for fish, mollusks, crustaceans, and aquatic mammals as well as the *OIE Manual of Diagnostic Tests and Vaccines for Terrestrial Animals* (*The Manual*) and a similar volume for aquatic animals. These manuals lay out validated diagnostic tests and vaccine production protocols.

The Code includes guidelines for disinfection and inactivation of the foot-and-mouth disease (FMD) virus and the causative agents of the transmissible spongiform encephalopathies (TSEs). There are also sections on transport of animals, surveillance systems, and notifiable diseases. *The Code* recommendations are intended to be trade-neutral. This means sanitary requirements should be the same for both importers and exporters.

The disease-specific standards in *The Code* vary in length and complexity depending on each disease's seriousness, mode of transmission, and the number of susceptible species. Disease chapters define each malady, the conditions required for disease-free status, and specific recommendations for international trade. Two diseases of major global concern, FMD and BSE, have the most detailed chapters.

The *OIE Code* also discusses diseases with similar and less complex guidelines than FMD or BSE. These are presented in eight groupings including: multiple species diseases (such as rabies and anthrax), cattle diseases, sheep and goat diseases, equine diseases, swine diseases, avian diseases, rabbit diseases, and bee diseases.

Countries may impose import measures that exceed *The Code* standards if they are scientifically justified and nondiscriminatory. If changes in import requirements are based on OIE standards, they don't have to be reported to the World Trade Organization.

OIE standards also include descriptions of diagnostic test methods and procedures for vaccine production and usage. These are published and regularly updated in the *OIE Manual*.

Relationships developed at OIE meetings help establish trust and lay the groundwork for international cooperation in livestock disease control and trade.

Other Related Organizations

In addition to the organizations described above, there are many other local, regional, national, and global veterinary organizations. These organizations represent many aspects of the practice of veterinary medicine as well as species and disciplinary specialties. Many of these are listed in the *AVMA Membership Directory & Resource Manual*[7] that is published every two years and can be found in the offices of most veterinarians.

These organizations present educational meetings which offer opportunities for veterinarians to communicate, come to agreement on current issues, and interact with other professions.

CHAPTER 12

CHALLENGES FACING VETERINARY MEDICINE

Introduction

Veterinary medicine—like most professions—faces dynamic and challenging changes in upcoming decades. If successful in your quest for admission to a college of veterinary medicine you will be affected, involved, and possibly expected to assume a leadership role in addressing issues facing the profession.

The fields of animal health and animal-related human health—like most other occupations—are undergoing changes that provide both opportunities and challenges. Before undertaking veterinary medicine, it is advisable to become familiar with some of these issues. It will require study to remain current and flexibility to adapt to changing technology. Some challenges facing the veterinary profession include:

- the rising costs of veterinary education;
- the positioning of veterinary medicine within academe;
- the management of zoonotic diseases;
- the control of exotic and emerging diseases;
- the rising costs of pet care;
- the increasing animal rights and humane concerns;
- the expanding veterinary knowledge base;
- the role of livestock health in world trade;
- the resistance of some animal diseases to eradication;
- the need for veterinarians in food animal medicine;
- the unique societal responsibilities of veterinarians; and
- the protection of the respected public image of the profession.

Each of these items will require organized and concerted efforts on the part of the profession and its members.

The Rising Costs of Veterinary Education

The complex costs of college education, for both students and their universities, continue to rise to levels that make many careers appear unachievable. Students can address this issue by scrimping and saving, dressing conservatively, buying only essential items, and eliminating spending on snacks and thus surviving the obesity epidemic. The cost of restaurant meals can be halved by drinking tap water and declining dessert. Packing a sandwich and not buying meals also saves considerable money.

There are many student jobs on college campuses. These include dining hall or restaurant jobs that provide meals, night librarian jobs, janitorial positions, landscaping work, assisting in laboratories, and many other income-generating opportunities. These jobs are usually not advertised and you have to ask to find them.

Part-time employment during vacations and weekends also helps reduce college debt. When you are working, you are not spending, so employment has two-fold financial benefits. Major rewards fall upon students who choose to work. Fellow students in college jobs can become lifelong companions. A wise course to follow is to sidestep financially and emotionally depleting habits associated with alcohol, tobacco, and drugs.

There are many scholarships available from hometown, state, and national organizations, and from on-campus sources. These can be accessed by a variety of routes that require effort and creativity. True financial need and academic achievement are required for some scholarships, but there are many other options.

The Positioning of Veterinary Medicine in Academe

The position of veterinary medicine in academic communities varies considerably among campuses. The cost per student to universities for veterinary students is among the highest of all disciplines. This results from the expense of multispecies clinical facilities and the added faculty needed for small-group clinical instruction. These factors place physical and financial limitations on veterinary class sizes.

The costs of veterinary education frequently raise the ire of university officials, curators, legislators, others with educational oversight responsibilities, as well as leaders of other academic disciplines. When these individuals learn the facts and become aware of the multiple contributions the profession makes to society, they generally understand.

In times of financial squeeze, this issue often resurfaces and requires diplomatic and articulate leadership to fend off efforts to close veterinary colleges or reduce their budgets. Opposition to cost-cutting proposals often comes from supporters of youth who are dreaming of being veterinarians and from members of the profession who depend on veterinary colleges for assistance and information.

There are a few anti-veterinary spokespersons in most states. This attitude can arise in individuals who applied for admission and were rejected by veterinary colleges despite good grades and high standard test scores; they might harbor resentment and disappointment, and blame the profession. Because repeatedly rejected applicants are often highly qualified, they can end up in high positions in industry, government, or academe, and they occasionally articulate their anti-veterinary opinions.

Increasing tuition costs, particularly for out-of-state residents, will be a long-term issue. The high cost per veterinary student is compounded by the number of years needed to achieve the training—in the form of residencies, internships, and advanced degrees—required to qualify for species and disciplinary specialties. The profession needs creative methods to address these challenges.

The Management of Zoonotic Diseases

Zoonotic diseases are animal diseases that are transmissible to people. Some human diseases that can be transmitted to animals are categorized as zoonoses because they originated in animals. Many zoonotic diseases are caused by bacteria. These include anthrax, brucellosis, cat scratch disease, leptospirosis, plague, salmonellosis, and tuberculosis.

Zoonoses caused by viruses include contagious ecthyma (orf), the equine encephalitides (Eastern, Western, St. Louis, and Venezuelan encephalitis, and West Nile disease), rabies, Rift Valley fever, vesicular stomatitis, and yellow fever. Many of the viral zoonoses, including equine viral infections, are transmitted by insect bites. Zoonotic diseases caused by fungi include actinomycosis, histoplasmosis, and ringworm.

You have probably heard about some zoonoses. By the time you've studied veterinary medicine for four years, they will all be familiar to you.

Federal and state surveillance systems are in place to monitor animal and human populations for zoonotic diseases. These systems are usually operated by organizations that focus on detection of exotic livestock diseases. All veterinarians, regardless of their career choice, are obligated to be alert for disease transmission from animals to humans and for possibilities of the introduction of zoonotic diseases.

The issue of zoonotic diseases is mutually addressed by the medical, nursing, veterinary, and public health professions. Few people recognize the magnitude of zoonotic diseases because many are transmittable from person-to-person and their animal origins become lost in the shuffle.

Public health workers provide governmental oversight and conduct activities that support the physical and mental well-being of communities. Actually, the veterinary profession, with its limited colleges and small cadre of graduates, does extremely well, especially considering the tiny number of colleagues directly involved in the control of zoonoses.

The management of diseases transmissible from animals to humans largely falls on state and federal public health officials who emphasize the human aspects of these diseases. The details of animal roles are largely taught in veterinary colleges, and only a small percentage of public health workers are veterinarians.

The Control of Exotic and Emerging Diseases

Exotic animal diseases are those that are absent from the USA. They are threats to US livestock and poultry populations that are currently free of them. This freedom provides competitive advantages to US agriculture. Emerging diseases are newly recognized diseases or diseases that are currently escalating in infectivity, virulence, or rapidity of spread.

Prolonged lack of exposure leaves US animal and poultry populations highly susceptible to exotic diseases and to many emerging diseases because they've never encountered their causative agents and have not been vaccinated. Thus they lack any immunity against them.

While vaccination might seem like a simple solution, it is not logical because vaccines are expensive, many must be repeated to be effective, and because animal populations are continually changing. These diseases often come in multiple strains which constantly mutate, and many are not preventable by available vaccines. In addition, the use of vaccines complicates their diagnosis because it is difficult to differentiate positive tests caused by natural infections from those induced by vaccination.

Every few years a new animal disease is recognized, identified, and named. Many of these also infect people. One emerging disease that receives much attention is bovine spongiform encephalopathy (BSE), a rare prion disease of cattle that causes the sometimes fatal Creutzfeldt-Jakob disease in man.

A currently emerging disease is human infection with swine influenza virus. Another still emerging disease is acquired immunodeficiency syndrome (AIDS) which is caused by the human immunodeficiency virus (HIV), and is believed to be of animal origin. AIDS-infected people are more likely to sicken when exposed to brucellosis, tuberculosis, and salmonellosis, parasitic infestations, and other animal diseases.

As the world's human populations multiply and closer human-to-human and human-to-animal contacts occur, these conditions will become more rampant, and specialized diagnostic and therapeutic procedures will be needed.

Among exotic livestock and poultry diseases, which are sometimes called foreign animal diseases, foot-and-mouth disease (FMD), BSE, and a poultry disease called exotic Newcastle disease (END) often receive media attention, but there are many other equally serious threats.

Foot-and-mouth disease (FMD) is a highly contagious viral infection of cattle, sheep, goats, swine, and numerous wildlife species. It is usually not fatal, but FMD virus infections are highly contagious and debilitating. They are among the most feared of animal health calamities.

FMD is characterized by an elevated temperature accompanied by rapidly rupturing painful vesicles (blisters) on the nose, mouth, tongue, and in the spaces between the claws of the hooves. These result in lameness, loss of appetite, and weight loss. There are multiple (and sometimes mutating) FMD virus strains that are prevalent in parts of Africa and South America. These foci of infection provide constant threats to the rest of the world.

When the FMD virus gains access to FMD-free countries, eradication is attempted by quarantine of affected regions, slaughter of infected animals, cleaning and disinfection of the premises, and cautious repopulation. This strategy and control of importation of animals and animal products helped the US to exclude FMD since 1929.

Bovine spongiform encephalopathy (BSE) is a slow-acting neurological disease of mature cattle. It is caused by ingestion of an abnormal protein (prion) that appears to be transmitted by feed contaminated by the meat or offal of BSE-infected cattle or small ruminants infected with scrapie. BSE was first recognized in Great Britain in an animal and human epidemic that lasted from 1986 to 1994.

BSE-infected mature cattle develop a variety of unusual behavioral patterns such as: incessant pacing; abnormally frequent water consumption and urination; lack of coordination; staggering; hanging of the head; weight loss; and a gradual decrease in appetite. BSE frequently terminates fatally due to aspiration of food into the lungs. BSE is usually diagnosed at postmortem exam by microscopic examination of the brain and testing for evidence of prions.

The human counterpart of BSE is Creutzfeldt-Jakob disease, a progressive and usually fatal condition that induces slowly appearing dementia, muscular twitching, blurred vision, and sleep disorders. It is suspected that this condition is transmitted by consumption of meat from BSE-infected cattle or scrapie-infected sheep.

Exotic Newcastle disease (END) is caused by highly pathogenic virus strains called virulent Newcastle disease viruses which are currently absent from the US. END is the objective of strict regulations and inspections imposed on the importation of poultry and pet birds into the US.

END was introduced into California poultry in 2002. It was finally eradicated in 2003, after an extensive and expensive program that involved quarantine and slaughter of all birds on infected and contact premises, and with carefully supervised repopulation.

The Rising Costs of Pet Care

The continually rising costs of pet ownership involve expensive pet foods that have replaced the formerly traditional diets of table scraps. There are also rising costs for the increasing number of vaccinations that become essential as more and more new diseases of pets are discovered and additional vaccines are developed. The rising costs of neutering procedures and other veterinary services result from the rising cost of living and increasing costs of continually improving surgical and anesthetic equipment.

These expenses are further stimulated by rapid advances in the understanding of the health and diseases of pet animals. This emerging knowledge has elevated the professional expectations for veterinarians to look more deeply into the details of each dog or cat they examine. This requires more time, additional tests, and expensive diagnostic procedures and equipment.

The emergence of group practices requires more money for salary and benefits, family support, and vacations for multiple practitioners that accomplish tasks formerly addressed by individual practitioners who worked 24/7, all year, for less money.

These comments must be attenuated by the reality that while veterinary education and specialty training programs are equally competitive and expensive to those of physicians, veterinary incomes are considerably lower than their medical colleagues and veterinary pharmaceuticals are often priced equally with human drugs.

The Increasing Animal Rights and Humane Concerns

There is a continually growing movement toward animal rights and increasing concerns about the humane treatment of livestock, pets, wildlife, and feral creatures (formerly domesticated animals living in the wild).

This movement reflects improved human virtue and adds new concerns and costs to the treatment and handling of animals. It also requires careful rethinking of procedures used in the medical and surgical treatment of pets, in the rearing and slaughtering of livestock and poultry, and in the use of animals in medical and pharmaceutical research.

The animal rights movement has continually pressured the veterinary profession to conform to their ideals, and many animal care and treatment procedures have been gradually modified to assure the utmost comfort for the animals and birds. These accommodations can be time-consuming and expensive, and their costs are passed on to consumers and clients.

The Expanding Veterinary Knowledge Base

There is an ever increasing quantity of veterinary knowledge due to new diseases, new infectious agents and parasites, and new diagnostic tests and equipment. The emergence of new specialties and techniques has expanded the profession's knowledge base. This expansion requires constant revision of the curriculums of veterinary colleges and added expenses for veterinary education.

In addition, there is a changing nature of how people look at animal diseases. This results from a combination of actual change, the emergence of new or previously unknown diseases, growing knowledge, and media attention attracted by recent international outbreaks of animal diseases.

The issues which the media chooses to feature can place a disproportionate emphasis on issues of minimal significance. As diagnostic and microbiologic technology advances, issues about the causes, methods of spread, and relationships with diet, travel, and vaccination become better understood, and the control and prevention of diseases become more complicated. These factors are enhanced by societal changes that diminish individual responsibility, so citizens rely on governments to solve problems while simultaneously accusing their leaders of excess spending.

The Role of Livestock Health in World Trade

The safety of foods and the health of livestock moved internationally are global concerns because of their economic risks. In addition to legitimate health and food safety issues, international trade issues are frequently raised to mask economic concerns of countries whose livestock and food industries are unable to compete with imported products.

There are legitimate dangers regarding the introduction of exotic human or animal diseases via animal or food importations. These concerns raise issues about identification of infected animals or products and traceability of the source of infections.

The control of international trade is complicated and controversial due to sheer numbers, frequent movement and transfer of livestock products and ownership, costs to government and animal owners, privacy, freedom of information, and international competitiveness.

The entity called the United States Department of Agriculture (USDA), Animal and Plant Health Inspection Service (APHIS), Veterinary Services (VS), National Center for Import and Export (NCIE) is entrusted with protecting US livestock and poultry from emerging and exotic diseases that might be introduced via legal or illegal entry of animals or animal products into the United States.

This responsibility is shared with the USDA Food Safety Inspection Service (FSIS) which is in charge of inspecting meat and poultry processing plants. The FSIS deals with foreign exporters and US importers and negotiates import-export requirements for foods of animal origin with representatives of other countries. They interact with trade alliances and strive to conform to guidelines and rules promulgated by the World Trade Organization (WTO) and the World Organization for Animal Health (OIE).

Foot-and-mouth disease (FMD), which is discussed above and also mentioned in chapter 11, is a highly communicable disease that infects many animal species. It is a prototype disease that is under continual discussion in international circles. A Hemispheric Conference on Eradication of FMD concluded that this disease—which affects ruminants and swine and can be transmitted by meat and by direct or indirect contact—is a threat to livestock health, international trade, and global prosperity. The Conference presented a long-range, strategic FMD eradication plan that includes:

- upgraded and accelerated surveillance;
- controlled movement of livestock and livestock products within and out of infected areas;
- expanded clinical and laboratory diagnosis;
- enforced quarantines and limits on human and vehicular movement out of infected areas;
- humane depopulation of infected and contact populations or mass vaccinations;
- cleaning and disinfection of premises; and
- supervised repopulation of formerly infected premises.

The Resistance of Some Animal Diseases to Eradication

Some animal diseases are remarkably resistant to eradication due to lifelong infections or unusually resistant infection agents.

The United States has faced prolonged and expensive challenges in its efforts to eradicate tuberculosis and brucellosis, two zoonotic diseases of US livestock. They both have been greatly reduced by federal-state cooperative disease control programs based on systematic testing, surveillance, animal movement controls, and in the case of brucellosis, by vaccination. They have not been completely eradicated for two reasons.

First, their ability to infect many species of animals as well as humans is challenging. There are foci of brucellosis-infected deer in Yellowstone Park and free-roaming, tuberculosis-infected deer in Michigan. Eliminating these infections would require massive slaughter of deer populations and these procedures are unacceptable to humane interests, wildlife support groups, and government wildlife agencies.

Second, both are caused by slow-growing, intracellular bacteria that are not easily eliminated from animal bodies by their immune systems or by antibacterial drugs. These organisms can be carried and transmitted by infected people or animals for years before the infected animals or people develop any signs of illness.

In the United States, animal disease eradication programs have succeeded in eliminating contagious bovine pleuropneumonia, FMD, hog cholera, vesicular exanthema, Venezuelan equine encephalitis, pullorum, and exotic Newcastle disease. The 2002–2003 outbreak of exotic Newcastle disease in poultry in California was successfully contained and then eradicated at the cost of millions of dollars.

The most efficient method of controlling exotic livestock and poultry diseases which exist throughout the world is the complex and costly process of preventing their introduction into countries where the diseases do not exist. Such programs require import control measures, surveillance, and testing.

The Need for Veterinarians in Food Animal Medicine

Sixty years ago veterinary medicine focused on general practice involving food animals, horses, and an occasional dog or cat.

In those days the ideal candidates for admission to veterinary colleges were bright young men who grew up on farms and thus were familiar with the feeding, care, and handling of various breeds of livestock.

Those statistics have changed. Now most aspiring DVMs are compassionate young women wishing to treat dogs or cats. Few applicants have farm backgrounds. As a result, colleges of veterinary medicine are searching for applicants with interests in food animal medicine.

The Unique Societal Responsibilities of Veterinary Medicine

Regardless of their career choices, all US veterinarians, by accepting a veterinary degree and swearing to the Veterinary Oath (see below), agree to undertake a set of unparalleled responsibilities that are unique to a profession whose members are singularly trained and exclusively qualified to accept them.

These responsibilities include serving as leaders in the veterinary aspects of public health and preserving the profession's public image by working and speaking with personal and professional honesty, sincerity, integrity, and credibility. Veterinarians in all walks of life are expected by friends, relatives, and acquaintances to be able to respond intelligently to queries about animal-disease-related issues which occasionally make headlines.

In this capacity, veterinarians serve as unique sources of knowledge and are experts and watchdogs of the public interest regarding zoonotic diseases, exotic diseases of animals, and the care and treatment of experimental animals in the specialty called laboratory animal medicine.

Preserving the Profession's Respected Public Image

The profession's respected public image is a precious legacy and a source of pride for all veterinarians. The vast majority of veterinarians appreciate the privilege of sharing the profession's reputation. They work to see that they add to its respectability. They also feel obligated to apologize for their mistakes, admit their limitations by referring challenging cases to specialists, and report the rare colleague who abuses the esteem of their profession.

The American Veterinary Medical Association (AVMA) has adopted the Veterinarian's Oath. It appears in each edition of the *AVMA Membership Directory & Resource Manual*[7], and many veterinary colleges administer this oath to each class at their graduation exercises. It goes like this:

> Being admitted to the profession of veterinary medicine, I solemnly swear to use my scientific knowledge and skills for the benefit of society through the protection of animal health, the relief of animal suffering, the conservation of animal resources, the promotion of public health, and the advancement of medical knowledge.
>
> I will practice my profession conscientiously and with dignity, and in keeping with the principles of veterinary medical ethics.

> I accept as a lifelong obligation the continual improvement of my professional knowledge and competence.

Conclusions about the Profession's Challenges

The challenges facing veterinary medicine include all those faced by professions requiring higher education. In addition, there are multiple issues that are distinct and unique to the profession.

These concerns, however, are not overwhelming, and other professions and employment opportunities each face their own specific problems. Therefore, these challenges, while essential to understanding the nature of the profession, should not dissuade aspiring veterinarians from pursuing their dreams.

CHAPTER 13

SO YOU STILL WANT TO BE A VETERINARIAN!

Introduction

After hearing about the challenges facing veterinarians and the number of applicants to veterinary colleges, you may be tempted to give up. Don't! There are many options open for those who choose to pursue this wonderful career.

If you have the personal determination, patience, and persistence to pursue these options, you can very well succeed in obtaining admission to a college of veterinary medicine and launching yourself into a rewarding career.

Multiple Challenges and Options

The challenges of veterinary medicine are not unique. Thus, suggestions about efficient use of youthful time and effort are applicable to most careers.

Until they mature physically and mentally, when it could appear to be—but actually isn't—too late, most people don't realize that success in this land of opportunity is not automatic. It requires passion, desire, and personal effort. Everyone has the potential to focus hard enough for these characteristics to emerge. Then, all that is needed is the persistence to implement them.

If nothing else, your passion for veterinary medicine and the inspiration to read this book will force a few decisions about how your years can be utilized. Decisions to invest youthful energy in preparing for competitive college admission procedures must come from within. In fact, they may actually be discouraged by parents or mentors. Nevertheless, recommendations from a third party who has experienced it (and is glad of it) might be followed. Let's hope this choice is true in your case.

Think twice before giving up on plans to participate in the profession of your dreams. It is filled with sincere, hardworking, and intelligent people who successfully overcame the same frustrations you may now be facing.

Don't Be Discouraged

If this book has discouraged you, please believe that was not its intention. It was designed to help you in the pursuit of a challenging and rewarding career. The book provides realistic descriptions of the challenges facing applicants to veterinary college and of the joys and rewards of the profession.

It also provides a touch of reality so that readers understand the challenges accompanying their ambition to become a doctor of veterinary medicine.

Some Alternatives

If you are pretty well convinced that you are not up to the challenges of attending a college of veterinary medicine or don't really want to go to college at all, consider some alternatives. First, store the idea of the veterinary career in the back of your mind—rather than completely abandoning it—and then proceed in another direction.

Try the military or get a job in an animal-related field. This could be at a kennel, on a farm, at a horse stable, at a zoo, or working for a veterinarian. After a few years of maturing and real-world experience, you may decide to reinvigorate your dream of being a veterinarian or decide to seek college-level training as a veterinary technologist or technician. These alternatives are described in chapter one.

Keep in mind that most veterinary colleges are striving for diversity in race, creed, color, national origin, age, and experience. They often make some admission decisions to help achieve those goals. Therefore, if you present a unique application as a mature student in your late twenties, you may find a spot in a college. The admission committees usually accept a couple of "senior citizens" in each class.

Conclusion

In conclusion, the advice suggested here arises from the author's actual experiences as a teenager in high school and as a pre-veterinary student in college. As a result of these experiences, I developed, expanded, and matured as a veterinary student, a practicing veterinarian, and as a faculty member who chaired a veterinary college admission committee. I hope this book has provided some useful insights.

Much of this information was learned the hard way or by observing friends and colleagues who would have been better off if they had read—and acted on—a book like this one when they were young.

If you follow the suggestions in *So You Want to Be a Veterinarian*, you might not realize it for some time, but eventually you will be glad you did. If you should choose to ignore them, you'll never know the difference but your career may be less rewarding and your life may be less satisfying.

If you launch a program to work your way through the challenges of a veterinary career, you won't be sorry and on graduation day you can proudly tell yourself that you knew all the time that you could do it.

Good luck and God bless you.

GLOSSARY

Words Defined as Used in Book)

AAVLD. See **American Association of Veterinary Laboratory Diagnosticians**.

AAVMC. See **Association of American Veterinary Medical Colleges**.

abscess. An inflamed cavity containing pus or other secretions that result from growth of bacteria. Abscesses often drain through passages to a surface.

academic specialties. Focused interests and knowledge involving an animal species or an academic discipline, usually attained by study and experience or by passing an examination.

accredited veterinary colleges. Colleges of veterinary medicine which are recognized by the Council on Education of the American Veterinary Medical Association as qualified to train veterinarians to practice in the United States after they complete state licensing requirements.

acetonemia. A non-febrile metabolic disease of mature, high-producing dairy cows in early stages of lactation (also called ketosis), caused by a deficiency of sugar and resulting in acetone in the blood and urine, and manifested by decreased appetite and reduced milk production. See also **ketosis**.

ACLAM. See **American College of Laboratory Animal Medicine**.

actinomycosis. A variety of human and animal abscess-like conditions, such as lumpy jaw of cattle, caused by infections with bacteria of the genus *Actinomyces*.

acquired immunodeficiency syndrome (AIDS). A chronic virus-induced human defect that gradually depletes the immune system's capacity to eliminate infections. It is transmitted by sexual intercourse and contact with body fluids and usually terminates fatally after a prolonged course.

acute mastitis. A bacterial infection of the bovine udder that is accompanied by inflammation, swelling, fever, reduced milk production, inappetence, and sometimes death.

admission. The process of granting or obtaining a position in a class at a college of veterinary medicine.

admission committees. Veterinary college committees, comprised mostly of faculty members, that design and administer the entry procedures.

admission requirements. The college courses, standard test scores, references, essays, and other criteria required for admission to veterinary colleges.

African horse sickness. An exotic, insect-transmitted, often fatal, equine viral disease that occurs in two forms (cardiovascular and respiratory) and is found in Africa and the Middle East.

African swine fever. An exotic, often fatal, porcine viral infection that is currently absent from the United States and can sometimes be confused with hog cholera.

AHI. See **Animal Health Institute**.

AIDS. See **acquired immunodeficiency syndrome**.

AJVR*.** See ***American Journal of Veterinary Research.

alopecia. Loss of hair.

alternate career choices. Veterinary careers other than the practice of veterinary medicine and treatment of animals.

American Association of Veterinary Laboratory Diagnosticians (AAVLD). An organization of veterinarians who are employed in diagnostic laboratories and who perform tests to determine the cause of animal ailments and/or deaths.

American College of Laboratory Animal Medicine (ACLAM). An organization that certifies veterinarians in the specialty of supervising the treatment and management of animals used in research.

American College Test (ACT). A standardized test that is used as an admission requirement by numerous colleges.

***American Journal of Veterinary Research* (*AJVR*).** A refereed journal published monthly by the AVMA. It contains reports on a variety of veterinary and animal-related research projects.

American Veterinary Medical Association (AVMA). The major United States all-purpose veterinary organization. It provides current information on veterinary issues and works to gain public and legislative support for the profession.

anal sacs. Small secretory glands located on each side of the anus of dogs. They sometimes become impacted or cancerous.

anatomic pathology. The study of the effects of disease and injuries on the structure and function of body parts.

anatomy. The study, description, and classification of the structure of body parts.

anesthesiology. The study of the products and procedures which reduce animal pain during medical manipulations or surgery.

animal behavior. The study of the habits, sometimes problematic, of animals that are often associated with aggressiveness or resistance to being housebroken, which are addressed by veterinarians and specialists who are referred to as animal behaviorists.

animal emergency centers. Veterinary hospitals that are open at night and on weekends and holidays to accommodate animal emergencies.

Animal Health Institute (AHI). An organization of corporations that manufacture and market animal health products like drugs, vaccines, and pesticides, and the members of government regulatory agencies that manage them.

anthelmintics. Drugs used to treat worm infestations.

anthrax. An often fatal febrile bacterial disease that can affect humans and most animal species and is usually acquired from contact with soil containing highly resistant spores of *Bacillus anthracis*.

antibiotics. Any of a wide variety of antimicrobial agents derived from living organisms that are used in the treatment of bacterial infections. They interfere with the reproduction of the causative agents. If not derived from living organisms, similar products are technically called antimicrobials.

antigens. Substances that the body recognizes as foreign and that invoke an immune response. Also, fractions of disease-producing agents that are used to invoke a recognizable response in testing for immunological reactions.

APHIS. The Animal and Plant Health Inspection Service. A US Department of Agriculture Agency responsible for preventing introduction of exotic animal and plant diseases into the United States.

aquatic animal medicine. The study of diseases of aquatic animals and the methods for their recognition, diagnosis, control, prevention, and treatment.

Association of American Veterinary Medical Colleges. (AAVMC). An organization housed in Washington, DC, that represents all the veterinary colleges in the US and Canada. It is run by the leadership of the academic community and represents the interests of veterinary education.

autopsy. Examination to determine the cause of human death. See also **necropsy**.

avian infectious laryngotracheitis. A globally distributed, often fatal, herpesvirus infection of chickens and pheasants that is characterized by inappetence, coughing, sniffling, and bloody nasal discharges.

avian influenza. An often mild infection of poultry, wild waterfowl, and psittacine (relating to parrots) birds. The virus can mutate to virulent forms called highly pathogenic avian influenza or fowl plague, which is exotic to the United States and invokes eradication efforts.

avian medicine. The study or practice of the diagnosis, prevention, and treatment of diseases of poultry and other bird species.

AVMA. See **American Veterinary Medical Association**.

AVMA Council on Education (COE). One of the elected councils of the AVMA. It inspects, evaluates, and accredits each US college of veterinary medicine.

AVMA Membership Directory & Resource Manual. An AVMA book that is published every two years. It lists the names and addresses of all members and officers, the membership of all AVMA councils, the AVMA rules and regulations, the code of veterinary ethics, and the names and addresses of most organizations that involve the veterinary profession.

bachelor's degree. The first and usually lowest degree conferred by four-year colleges or universities. It usually requires the equivalent of four years of college-level studies.

bacteria. Small single-celled microorganisms that can infect animals and people, causing diseases. Bacteria can survive and multiply in the environment.

bacteriology. The study of the classification, structure, functions, and recognition of bacteria and the diseases they cause.

barking pig syndrome. See **Nipah virus**.

biochemistry. The chemistry of living organisms and the many life processes of humans, animals, and other living things.

biopsy. A diagnostic procedure involving removal and examination of tissues, cells, or fluids from a live animal's body to determine the cause of a problem.

bloat. Gaseous and potentially fatal distention of the gastrointestinal tract, most commonly the fourth stomach (rumen) of ruminants.

board certification. A process for certifying veterinarians as having the required skills and experience in certain specialties, achieved by training and sometimes examination.

bottle jaw. An edematous swelling below the jaw of worm-infested ruminants.

bovine medicine. The branch of veterinary medicine that deals with the description, diagnosis, treatment, control, and prevention of diseases and disorders of cattle.

bovine myxovirus parainfluenza-3 (BPI-3). A bovine virus which, when triggered by stress and bacterial complications, produces a highly infectious febrile disease called "shipping fever."

bovine spongiform encephalopathy (BSE). A prion-produced, contagious, but slow-spreading, chronic zoonotic infection of cattle that causes a spongy degeneration of brain tissue and abnormal behavioral patterns. It is probably acquired by consumption of bone meal or other tissues of sheep that are infected with scrapie and is probably transmitted to people by eating beef from infected cattle.

bovine viral diarrhea (BVD). A sometimes fatal viral infection of cattle that produces fever, diarrhea, and erosions of the mucous membranes of the mouth and can produce a chronic carrier state in calves of cows infected during pregnancy. Some BVD infections are mild and unobserved.

brucellosis. Zoonotic infections caused by intracellular bacteria of the genus *Brucella* that produce abortion and other reproductive disorders in cattle (*B. abortus);* swine (*B. suis*); sheep and goats (*B. Miletensis*); and dogs (*B. canis*). Human infections are often called undulant fever or Malta fever. They are characterized by fever, widespread pain, and weakness.

BSE. See **bovine spongiform encephalopathy**.

bursa. A sac or closed cavity, often (but not necessarily) located between tendons and bones, the internal lining of which secretes fluids that cushion the movements of body parts. See also **bursal disease**.

bursal disease. An immunosuppressive, contagious viral disease of chickens often manifested by diarrhea, neurologic disorders, and swelling of the cloacal bursa.

calculi. Plural of calculus: small abnormal stones or gelatinous plugs formed by mineral accumulations, usually found in the urinary tract or bile ducts.

calf scours. Diarrhea in calves.

canine distemper. A highly contagious canine viral infection which causes fever, loss of appetite, runny nose, ocular discharge, and a variety of other disorders, including nervous signs which may follow apparent recovery.

canine hepatitis. A sometimes fatal, contagious viral infection of dogs and some wild species, that causes fever, depression, prolonged clotting time, and sometimes internal hemorrhages and enlargement of the liver. It is often followed by a corneal opacity.

canine medicine. The branch of veterinary medicine that deals with the description, diagnosis, treatment, prevention, and control of diseases and disorders of dogs.

canine parvovirus. A fecal-borne canine virus which can cause diarrhea, vomiting, fever, and, rarely, inflammation of the heart muscle.

caprine. Related to goats.

caprine arthritis-encephalitis. A viral infection of goats which causes unobserved infections and sometimes debilitating arthritis.

cardiology. The study of the anatomy, physiology, and normal functions of the heart and the diagnosis, treatment, prevention, and control of cardiac diseases and disorders.

cardiovascular. Dealing with the heart and blood circulation.

caseous lymphadenitis. A disease shared by sheep and goats and occasionally by people. It is characterized by slow-growing, painful abscesses throughout the body and is caused by a bacterium called *Salmonella pseudotuberculosis*.

CAST. See **Council for Agricultural Science and Technology**.

cat-scratch disease. A human bacterial skin infection at the site of wounds inflicted by the bites or the scratches of cats, and characterized by short-lived blisters, swelling of local lymph nodes, and fever.

Chief Veterinary Officer. The highest-ranking veterinarian in a nation's government who serves as the country's delegate to the World Organisation for Animal Health (OIE).

chlamydia. A specialized genus of intracellular bacteria that causes avian psittacosis and eye, intestinal, or brain infections in several species.

classical swine fever. See **hog cholera**.

clinical. Dealing with observable disease manifestations and the hands-on examination and treatment of animals.

clinical pathology. The practice of the diagnosis of diseases, usually based on the history, clinical signs, and a variety of laboratory tests and procedures.

clinical practice. The practice of veterinary medicine with a focus on the examination and treatment of live animals.

cloacal bursa. The mucus-secreting sac that surrounds the posterior opening of poultry and birds.

coccidiosis. A parasitic infestation of the gastrointestinal tract of livestock, which causes diarrhea and weight loss and is occasionally fatal. It is common in confined animals.

COE. See **AVMA Council on Education**.

colic. A name for painful gastrointestinal disorders of horses.

coliforms. Bacteria of the *Escherichia coli* species that inhabit the intestinal tract of humans and most animals and occasionally cause disease.

companion animal medicine. The practice of veterinary medicine on companion animals, which are mostly dogs and cats.

companion animals. Pets and animals kept as companions, usually dogs and cats.

contagious ecthyma. A contagious virus-induced skin infection of sheep and goats that causes papules, vesicles, and eventually scabs on the mouth, udder, and sometimes on the feet of young animals. It results in loss of appetite and ultimately in weight loss. It can be partially prevented by vaccination.

corneal opacity. An opaque white discoloration of the usually clear front portion of the eye (the cornea).

corporate careers. Veterinary careers working with companies or corporations such as pharmaceutical manufacturers or dog food producers.

corporate practices. Officially incorporated veterinary practices, usually with multiple veterinarians.

Council for Agricultural Science and Technology (CAST). An organization of scientific societies and individuals that prepares task force reports and issues papers. CAST documents contain scientifically accurate information in formats understandable to the general public.

Council on Biological and Therapeutic Agents. An elected council that advises the AVMA Executive Board about issues, positions, and guidelines for the development, production, and use of drugs and vaccines for diagnosing, preventing, and treating diseases of animals.

Council on Education (COE). An elected council which advises the AVMA Executive Board about accrediting colleges of veterinary medicine.

Council on Public Health and Regulatory Veterinary Medicine. An elected council that advises the AVMA Executive Board about positions and guidelines for development and use of policies regarding public health and regulatory veterinary medicine.

credibility. A favorable reputation regarding professional honesty, trustworthiness, reliability, and believability.

curriculums. The required and elective courses of study available in colleges of veterinary medicine.

CVM. College of veterinary medicine.

CVO. See **Chief Veterinary Officer**.

Dale Carnegie Course. A series of courses presented in many locations, which offers instruction in public speaking and interpersonal relations as espoused by Dale Carnegie.

dermatology. The study of skin, its anatomy and physiology, and the treatment of its diseases.

diagnosis. The identification of the nature and cause of health problems by coordinated examination of the history, clinical signs, and antemortem and postmortem lesions of affected animals.

diaphragm. The dome-shaped muscular partition that separates the abdominal and thoracic cavities.

differential diagnosis. The list of possible causes of infection and other ailments, which is narrowed by additional observations and test results.

diplomate. A title assigned to a specialist who has completed all the requirements of a specialty organization.

discipline specialties. Veterinary specialties developed through training in medical techniques in areas like surgery, radiology, and ophthalmology.

distemper. A broad term indicating a number of physical disorders, usually assigned to viral infections characterized by fever, nasal discharge, and inappetence. See also **canine**, **feline**, and **equine distemper**.

diversity. Population variety with respect to age, gender, race, creed, color, and national origin.

Doctor of Veterinary Medicine (DVM). The academic degree awarded after four years of study in all US colleges of veterinary medicine except the University of Pennsylvania, which grants the Veterinary Medical Doctor (VMD) degree.

DVM. See **Doctor of Veterinary Medicine**.

DVM degree. The Doctor of Veterinary Medicine degree granted upon graduation after four years of study at all US veterinary colleges except the University of Pennsylvania, which grants the Veterinary Medical Doctor (VMD) degree.

Eastern equine encephalomyelitis. A mosquito-borne virus infection of Western Hemisphere horses that infects wild birds and poultry as well as people, causing a wide variety of neurologic signs.

ECFVG. See **Educational Commission for Foreign Veterinary Graduates**.

edema. Abnormal accumulation of fluid in tissues.

edema disease. A highly fatal infection that affects healthy, recently weaned piglets. It is caused by certain strains of *Escherichia coli* bacteria and is manifested by edema of gastrointestinal organs and subcutaneous tissues. See also **gut edema** or **bowel edema**.

Educational Commission for Foreign Veterinary Graduates (ECFVG). An AVMA certification program for graduates of nonaccredited foreign veterinary colleges that qualifies them for application for state veterinary licenses based on English language proficiency, scientific knowledge, and hands-on skills.

emergency medicine. The phase of medicine or veterinary medicine that deals with emergencies.

encephalitides. The plural form of the word encephalitis.

encephalitis. Inflammation of the brain.

epidemiology. The study of the distribution, incidence, and the prevalence of diseases in populations, and the development of preventive and control measures based on data and observations.

epididymis. A coiled duct that transmits sperm out of the testicles.

epididymitis. Inflammation or injury to the epididymis.

epidural. An anesthetic procedure used to prevent animals in labor from straining, to permit manipulation of the fetus and expedite safe delivery. It is accomplished by injecting local anesthetics between the spinal bones of the tail.

equine distemper. See **strangles**.

equine encephalitides. The collective name for the several virus infections that cause encephalitis of horses. See also **Eastern equine encephalomyelitis** and **Western equine encephalitis**.

equine infectious anemia. An insect-transmitted viral infection of horses that manifests a gamut of signs, from mild, unobserved infections to a severe and sometimes fatal anemia.

equine influenza. A rapidly spreading, viral respiratory disease of horses that produces fever, nasal discharge, cough, and severe depression. The incidence can be reduced by vaccination and isolation.

equine medicine. The study and practice dealing with the diagnosis, treatment, prevention, and control of diseases of horses.

equine rhinopneumonitis. A herpesvirus infection of horses that causes relatively mild respiratory disease and abortion.

equine viral abortion. Equine abortion caused by herpesviruses similar to those causing equine viral rhinopneumonitis.

equine viral arteritis. An acute, rapidly spreading, viral infection of horses that produces fever, depression, edematous swellings of the skin, and sometimes nasal and ocular discharge or abortion.

ethics. See ***Principles of Veterinary Medical Ethics***.

exotic Newcastle disease. A globally distributed avian virus infection that causes mild or unobserved respiratory infections. It also has highly virulent mutations that can induce fatal infections and occasional neurologic disorders. These virulent strains require eradication.

extension. An outreach component of academic communities charged to deliver information to the public via websites, printed documents, meetings, and public speaking engagements.

extracurricular activities. Nonacademic programs, such as band, chorus, debate, and sports, undertaken voluntarily by students at schools and colleges.

febrile diseases. Diseases characterized by fever.

feline distemper. A globally distributed viral infection of cats that produces a variety of vague and often mild signs, plus weight loss, depression, and severe inflammation of internal organs. See also **feline panleukopenia**.

feline infectious peritonitis. A usually mild or unobserved viral infection that can occasionally produce fatal neurologic and/or abdominal infections.

feline leukemia. An often fatal viral infection of cats that results in tumors, anemia, and immunologic deficiencies, and is also called feline lymphoma and feline lymphosarcoma.

feline medicine. The study and practice of the diagnosis, treatment, control, and prevention of diseases of cats.

feline panleukopenia. An acute, sometimes fatal, viral infection of young kittens and cats that often causes only a mild depression. When severe, it produces fever, dehydration, diarrhea, and vomiting.

feline pneumonitis. A slightly erroneous name for chlamydial conjunctivitis, which is a feline bacterial infection that causes runniness of the eyes.

fetal presentation. The part of the fetus that attempts to emerge first during birth. In anterior presentation the head and/or the front legs appear, and in posterior presentation the hind legs emerge. In a breech presentation, the rear end emerges with the hind legs extended forward and adjustment is required.

fistula. An abnormal opening between internal organs and body surfaces or between two internal body organs, that permits passage of material between the two.

float. A file with a foot-long handle used to file horses' teeth. See **floating teeth**.

floating teeth. The filing of a horse's teeth to blunt sharp edges.

FMD. See **foot-and-mouth disease**.

foci. Plural form of the word focus. See also **focus**.

focus. The central location from which an infection or malignancy originates.

Food Safety Inspection Service (FSIS). A regulatory agency of the US Department of Agriculture that is charged with protecting the safety of food.

foot-and-mouth disease (FMD). A highly contagious disease of cattle, swine, sheep, and goats caused by multiple and rapidly mutating virus strains. It causes rupturing blisters on an animal's feet and mouth, fever, depression, lameness, loss of appetite, and weight loss. It would spread rapidly through countries that are currently free of the disease if it gained access to them.

foot rot. A bacterial infection of the space between the claws of ruminants, that causes lameness.

fowl plague. Another name for avian influenza.

FSIS. See **Food Safety Inspection Service**.

general practice. A veterinary practice that addresses the needs of all animal species.

GIVE. See **Global Initiatives in Veterinary Education**.

Global Initiatives in Veterinary Education (GIVE). A cooperative program of the Association of American Veterinary Medical Colleges that creates partnerships between US veterinary colleges and veterinary colleges in developing countries to strengthen veterinary education.

graduate education. Advanced collegiate studies undertaken after graduation from four-year college programs, that usually result in an MS or a PhD degree.

Graduate Record Examination (GRE). One of the standard tests administered to college students to assess their academic fitness for collegiate graduate studies.

grant overhead. Governmental payments to universities to help cover the infrastructural costs incurred by implementation of federal projects and grants.

GRE. See **Graduate Record Examination**.

group practice. A veterinary practice comprised of three or more veterinarians.

gut edema. Another name for contagious ecthyma. See also **orf**, **sore mouth**, and **contagious ecthyma**.

hardware. The common name for nails, screws, or wire scraps that may litter farmlands and produce traumatic peritonitis, which results when the items are swallowed by cattle and penetrate the cow's gastrointestinal tract, causing debilitating internal infections.

hardware disease. See **hardware**.

herpesviruses. A large group of viruses which infect all species of animals and humans, causing a variety of diseases characterized by permanent, inactive infections which can later be reactivated by stress and provide sources of infections for susceptible individuals.

higher education. Educational programs undertaken after high school.

histology. The microscopic study of anatomy.

histopathology. The microscopic study of the effects of disease and injury on tissues and organs.

histoplasmosis. A globally distributed, chronic fungal infection of people, dogs, cats, and other animals. It is most common in river valleys and produces a wide variety of clinical signs including lymph node enlargement and sometimes death. The causative agent, *Histoplasma capsulatum*, survives in soil.

HIV. See **human immunodeficiency virus**.

hog cholera. A highly contagious and often fatal viral disease of swine, characterized by fever, loss of appetite, diarrhea, and death. It is also called classical swine fever and is presently eradicated from the United States.

HSUS. See **Humane Society of the United States**.

human immunodeficiency virus (HIV). The viral cause of acquired immunodeficiency syndrome (AIDS), a human disease causing fatigue, loss of appetite, chills, intermittent fever, susceptibility to multiple infections, and premature death.

Humane Society of the United States (HSUS). A nationally prominent organization dedicated to the humane care and treatment of animals.

IBR. See **infectious bovine rhinotracheitis**.

infectious bovine rhinotracheitis (IBR). A viral infection of cattle, characterized by fever, respiratory distress, abortion, and subsequent latent infections subject to stress-induced reactivations.

infectious bronchitis. A viral-induced upper respiratory infection of chickens, characterized by coughing, sneezing, reduced egg production, and slow growth rates.

infectious canine hepatitis. A globally distributed viral disease of dogs and most other canine animals, characterized by fever, reduced appetite, edema of the skin around the head and neck, and, often, spotty hemorrhages in the gastrointestinal tract. After recovery, a corneal opacity often develops in one eye.

integrity. Honesty, sincerity, and dedication to the principles of veterinary ethics.

internal medicine. Medical or veterinary procedures involving internal organs and ailments which cannot be seen visually.

***International Animal Health Code* (*The Code*).** A code prepared and updated by the World Organisation for Animal Health that outlines guidelines for safe international movement of animals and animal products.

interns. Veterinarians undertaking the initial year of advanced training for specialties.

internships. Positions providing the initial year of advanced training for specialties.

JAVMA*.** See ***Journal of the American Veterinary Medical Association.

***Journal of the American Veterinary Medical Association* (*JAVMA*).** A professional journal with items of veterinary interest published twice monthly by the AVMA and distributed to its members.

ketones. Sweet-smelling bodily substances resembling acetone which arise when inadequate glucose is available as a source of energy. Present in bovine ketosis.

ketosis. See **acetonemia**.

laboratory animal medicine. That branch of veterinary medicine which deals with the care and use of research animals.

laboratory animals. Animals used for research purposes.

large animal practice. Veterinary practices involving horses or farm animals.

leptospira pomona. A spiral-shaped bacterium of the genus *Leptospira* that survives in urine, infects cattle, horses, and swine (sometimes causing abortion), and occasionally infects humans and other species.

leptospirosis. A worldwide urine-transmitted bacterial infection of the kidneys that affects most animal species (including humans) and causes fever and sometimes abortion.

lesions. Abnormalities or changes in body tissues or organs.

liver flukes. Parasites that invade the liver of sheep, causing serious disease, and that infest cattle with minimal damage. They are usually acquired by invasive portions of the parasite.

lungworms. A variety of parasitic infestations of the lower airways as a result of infestation by several species of worm parasites.

lymph nodes. Small, oval-shaped organs widely distributed in animal and human bodies, that produce disease-fighting cells (lymphocytes), and an immunologically active liquid (lymph) which circulates through the body to fight infections.

malpractice. Professional negligence or failure to exercise reasonable judgment in professional decisions.

Marek's disease. A highly fatal, globally distributed herpesvirus infection of turkeys and chickens. Clinical disease is absent in many infected flocks.

Master of Science degree (MS). A postgraduate college degree that is usually awarded after two years of study following receipt of the bachelor's degree and completion of a thesis and an examination.

melioidosis. A chronic bacterial infection causing abscesses in a variety of bodily locations. It is present in some parts of Asia and Australia. It infects humans and most animal species via contact with contaminated soil.

mentors. Teachers, coaches, or informed advisors.

metritis. Inflammation of the uterus.

microbiology. The study of microorganisms.

milk bag. See **udder**.

mixed practice. A veterinary practice that deals with multiple species of animals.

MS degree. The collegiate graduate degree called a Master of Science.

mucosa. Thin tissues that line body parts that open to the outside, such as the digestive, respiratory, reproductive, and urinary tracts, and that sometimes produce mucus. See also **mucous membranes**.

mucous membranes. See **mucosa**.

NAFV. See **National Association of Federal Veterinarians**.

NAP. See **National Academies of Practice**.

NASULGC. See **National Association of State Universities and Land Grant Colleges**.

National Academies of Practice (NAP). A multidisciplinary US medical organization that includes physicians, veterinarians, dentists, nurses, and other health professions; it works to educate the public and legislators about health issues of national significance.

National Association of Federal Veterinarians (NAFV). An organization that represents veterinarians employed by the federal government.

National Association of State Universities and Land Grant Colleges (NASULGC). An organization of administrative officials of US state universities which meets annually to develop policies and positions supporting higher education. It lobbies legislators and prepares documentation of academic needs.

National Association of Veterinary Technicians in America (NAVTA). An organization of veterinary assistants, technicians, and technologists, that works to maintain high standards in animal care.

National Institute for Animal Agriculture (NIAA). A national organization of livestock producers, regulators, veterinarians, and scientists, that represents organizational, corporate, governmental, and academic interests, and provides forums for developing issues concerning animal agriculture.

NAVTA. See **National Association of Veterinary Technicians in America**.

NIAA. See **National Institute for Animal Agriculture**.

necropsy. A postmortem examination to determine the cause of animal deaths.

nephrology. The study of normal and abnormal kidney function.

neurology. The study of the normal and abnormal structure and function of the nervous system.

Newcastle disease. A usually mild but rapidly mutating, globally distributed viral respiratory, gastrointestinal, and neurological infectious disease of poultry and wild birds.

NGO. Nongovernmental organization.

Nipah virus. A bat-transmitted viral infection of swine, sometimes called "barking pig syndrome," that produces fever, coughing, and respiratory distress. It occasionally infects people working closely with pigs and produces human encephalitis.

non-practice activities. Veterinary activities that are conducted by veterinarians but do not involve hands-on treatment of animals.

nontenured appointments. Academic appointments with nonprofessorial titles and lacking the job security granted to tenured faculty members.

nutrition. The processes of intake, absorption, assimilation, and use of food and nutrients.

offal. By-products or trimmings, including the viscera of butchered animals, which are often used in animal feeds.

OIE. The Office International des Épizooties, now called the World Organisation for Animal Health, while retaining its original abbreviation (OIE).

ophthalmology. The branch of medicine dealing with the structure, function, and disorders of the eyes.

orchitis. Inflammation of the testicles.

orf. A contact-transmitted poxvirus infection of sheep and goats which produces papules, pustules, and vesicles on the lips, mouth, and feet. It is also called sore mouth and contagious pustular dermatitis.

overhead. See **grant overhead**.

overhead dollars. Funds accessed, usually as a percentage, by universities on incoming grant dollars to cover the added infrastructural costs required by the funded project.

ovine. Dealing with sheep.

PAHO. See **Pan American Health Organization**.

palpation. Manual touching and feeling during a physical examination to determine the size, shape, location, and other characteristics of organs, tumors, or fetuses.

Pan American Health Organization (PAHO). An international organization that promotes health throughout the Americas by holding dialog among decision makers, educators, and other organizations to ensure that health programs are available to all.

papules. Small, solid, raised areas on the skin, usually less than one centimeter in diameter.

parasites. Organisms that live on or inside other organisms and obtain their nourishment from their host, sometimes causing disruptions to host functions.

parasitology. The branch of medical science that focuses on the identification, prevention, and control of parasites and the diseases they cause.

parturition. The process of giving birth.

pathology. The study of the identification, description, recognition, causes, and effects of diseases by analysis of the structure and the function of body parts.

pericardium. A membranous sac, containing small amounts of fluid, that surrounds the heart.

peritoneum. The membrane that lines the walls of the abdominal cavity and covers the surface of abdominal organs.

peritonitis. Inflammation of the peritoneum, usually by bacteria, that results in abdominal pain and sometimes death.

pharmacology. The study of the properties, actions, uses, doses, and antidotes of drugs.

PhD. An abbreviation for Doctor of Philosophy, the highest academic degree.

physiology. The study of the structural and biochemical processes and the functional mechanisms of the body and its parts.

placenta. The uterine appendage (fetal sac) that surrounds the fetus and provides its circulation and nutrition during pregnancy. It is normally expelled at parturition. See also **retained placenta**.

plague. Any deadly epidemic disease, more specifically a flea-transmitted, human infection caused by the bacteria called *Yersinia pestis*.

porcine. Dealing with pigs.

porcine tuberculosis. Tuberculosis in pigs, which causes widespread lymph node enlargement and can result from infection with avian, bovine, or human *tubercle bacilli.*

practice specialties. Species and disciplinary areas of expertise and focus, which require a unique knowledge, skill, and experience to establish veterinarians as specialists and experts.

practitioners. Veterinarians involved with hands-on animal care.

presentation. See **fetal presentation**.

preventive/preventative medicine. The disciplinary specialty (also known as herd health) that involves comprehensive programs designed to reduce or eliminate animal diseases through vaccinations, environmental stabilization, isolation, nutritional excellence, and disease control programs.

pre-veterinary requirements. Collegiate-level coursework required for application to colleges of veterinary medicine.

Principles of Veterinary Medical Ethics. A code of ethics that is published in the *AVMA Membership Directory & Resource Manual*. The code outlines desired professional ethics, behavior, and practices.

prions. Tiny atypical intracellular particles that cause neurologic diseases like BSE and scrapie.

private practices. Veterinary practices that are owned and operated by individual veterinarians as opposed to employment by academic, government, or corporate organizations.

private practitioners. Self-employed veterinarians that work independently or in groups.

proceedings books. The recorded and distributed summaries of presentations delivered at meetings.

professional ethics. Moral values or standard behaviors that are expected of veterinarians.

prolapse. See **prolapsed uterus**.

prolapsed uterus. An exteriorization of the uterus through the vagina following birth of newborns. A prolapse comprises an emergency that requires immediate veterinary attention.

public health. The field of human medicine focused on the health of communities by addressing issues like vaccinations, food and water safety, zoonotic diseases, pollution, waste disposal, and environmental and workplace health.

public practice. The practice of veterinary medicine while in the employment of governmental agencies.

pullorum disease. An egg-transmitted bacterial infection of chickens and turkeys, caused by *Salmonella pullorum*, and which causes high mortality in young birds.

pus. The white, creamy fluid comprising mostly white blood cells and necrotic debris resulting from localized bacterial infections.

rabies. A usually fatal, bite-transmitted, viral infection of mammals, with reservoirs in bats and numerous wildlife species. Companion animals require rabies vaccination.

radiology. The study and use of radiation, X-rays, or radioactive materials in the diagnosis and treatment of disease.

referrals. Suggestions that clients have their animals examined by another veterinarian or a specialist.

regulatory activities. Programs assuring that activities are in compliance with laws and regulations.

regulatory careers. Employment by government agencies that conduct regulatory activities.

residencies. Two-year periods of advanced study and experience in post-DVM training for specialties, usually partaken after an internship is completed.

residents. Participants in residency programs.

retained placenta. Failure of the placenta to be delivered with a fetus at parturition, and a condition often requiring veterinary intervention. See also **placenta**.

reticulum. The most forward of the stomachs of ruminant animals into which the esophagus empties swallowed food.

rickettsia. A genus of infectious microorganisms with some characteristics of both bacteria and viruses, that are often transmitted by rodents.

rickettsial diseases. Diseases caused by *rickettsia*, including human Rocky Mountain spotted fever and animal diseases like Q fever, eperythrozoonosis, ehrlichiosis, murine typhus, and rickettsial pox. See also **rickettsia**.

Rift Valley fever. An acute mosquito-borne viral infection of ruminants that is transmissible to humans when they are closely associated with infected animals. Endemics occur periodically in eastern Africa and on the Arabian Peninsula. It is currently exotic to North America.

ringworm. The common name for a number of crusty or scaly (sometimes itchy) fungal infections of the skin of animals and people. It is often accompanied by hair loss in circular patterns.

rumen. The largest of the four stomachs of ruminant animals.

ruminants. Cud-chewing, even-toed, hoofed animals including goats, sheep, cattle, deer, camels, and giraffes.

salmonellosis. Infection of animals or people with bacteria of the genus *Salmonella*, usually acquired due to contaminated foods or direct or indirect contact with infected feces; often involving the gastrointestinal tract, sometimes without clinical signs and sometimes causing a severe gastroenteritis.

SAT. See **Scholastic Aptitude Test**.

Scholastic Aptitude Test. A standardized test administered to students in high school to evaluate their qualifications for college.

scrapie. A chronic, slowly developing, eventually fatal, nervous disease of sheep, characterized by incoordination and a variety of behavioral changes, and probably caused by prions or similar particles.

sepsis. Infection of wounds or tissues with bacteria, or multiplication of bacteria in the blood. See also **septicemia**.

septicemia. Infection of the blood with bacteria and their toxins.

serology. A branch of microbiology that evaluates blood serum for evidence of diseases.

serum. Clear, watery body fluids including cell-free blood.

signs. Manifestations of disease or injury as seen by observers like veterinarians or physicians. Compare with **symptoms**.

small animal practice. A veterinary practice involving mostly pets.

small animal surgery. The study and performance of corrective manipulation or operative procedures on tissues or organs of companion animals.

sore mouth. Another name for contagious ecthyma or orf in sheep or goats.

specialties. Unique practice qualifications, usually in a certain discipline or animal species, acquired by advanced training and experience and sometimes requiring examinations for recognition as a specialist.

specialty boards and specialty colleges. Organizations of veterinary experts that provide recognition of qualified veterinarians as specialists and offer continuing education programs and sometimes require examinations for membership.

specialty organizations. Organizations of veterinary specialists.

species specialties. Veterinary specialties that focus on the diagnosis, prevention, treatment, and control of diseases of a certain species.

standard test scores. The results of examinations that are taken by high school or college students to qualify for admission to college programs. See also **SAT** and **GRE**.

state board examinations. Written and/or practical examinations administered to veterinarians, usually recent graduates, to qualify them to become state licensed veterinarians.

state work. Veterinary services contracted to practitioners by state disease control programs, often involving brucellosis and tuberculosis programs.

stiff lamb disease. A sometimes fatal neuromuscular degeneration of neonatal lambs, caused by a deficiency of selenium and vitamin E. See also **white muscle disease**.

St. Louis encephalitis. A mosquito-transmitted virus infection of wild and domestic birds that can cause encephalitis in humans bitten by infected insects.

strangles. An acute infection of horses caused by *Streptococcus equi* that produces fever, depression, nasal discharge, and a swelling of the lymph nodes in the throat. It often appears in assembled or recently transported horses. Often called **equine distemper**.

summer sores. Infestations of horses with larvae of stomach worms that are deposited on existing cuts or sores by flies. The condition is also called cutaneous habronemiasis.

surgery. The branch of veterinary medicine that addresses conditions that require manipulation or operations for their correction.

swine erysipelas. A sometimes fatal bacterial infection of pigs, characterized by fever, reluctance to move, and purple discoloration of the skin.

swine vesicular disease. An infectious viral disease of pigs, which can resemble foot-and-mouth disease because both can cause eruptions of the skin of the nose, mouth, and feet.

symptoms. The feelings or perceptions of the effects of disease or injuries as described by human patients. Compare to **signs**.

syndrome. A collection of clinical signs with a common cause.

tenure. A permanent job appointment in academe that awards professorial titles to faculty who have demonstrated scholarly productivity in their field of specialization.

theriogenology. The professional study of animal reproduction.

Toastmasters International. A nonprofit organization with almost 12,000 clubs throughout the world and over 230,000 members, that provides support for people interested in improving their public speaking skills and interpersonal relations. Members positively critique each others' talks and suggest improvements.

toxicology. The study of poisonous substances, their effects, their diagnosis, and their treatments in various species.

trichinosis. Human infestations with the larvae of *Trichinella spiralis*, acquired by eating undercooked pork. Some infestations can be asymptomatic, others are serious.

trocar. A sharp-pointed rod that fits inside a tube called a cannula, to pierce body cavities and permit escape of gas or fluids, after removal of the pointed trocar.

tuberculosis. A group of chronic infections by various species of specific tuberculosis bacteria of animals and man. These produce widespread, tumor-like granular nodules in the lungs and throughout the body. Unless treated, TB can terminate fatally.

udder. Bag-like milk-producing organs of cows and other animals.

USAHA. See **US Animal Health Association**.

US Animal Health Association (USAHA). An association of animal health organizations and individuals dedicated to stabilizing and improving the health of US and global livestock populations.

vesicle. A small blister containing clear fluid.

vesicular exanthema. A highly contagious porcine viral infection characterized by blisters on the feet, nose, and mouth.

vesicular stomatitis. A viral infection affecting cattle, horses, swine, and occasionally sheep or goats in the Western Hemisphere. It is characterized by excessive salivation and development of rapidly rupturing vesicles and ulcers in the mouth or on the feet and teats, resembling mild cases of foot-and-mouth disease.

Veterinarian's Oath. A declaration and promise to practice the profession with high ethical standards and with professional credibility and personal integrity.

veterinary assistants. Veterinary employees who perform functions requiring minimal professional training, sometimes without formal technician training. See also **veterinary technicians** or **veterinary technologists**.

Veterinary Medical College Application Service (VMCAS). A preliminary step in application to veterinary colleges. This service is managed by the Association of American Veterinary Medical Colleges. It scans applications for evidence that applicants have completed all required courses, standardized tests, and other requirements.

veterinary curriculums. The courses of study for the DVM or VMD degrees offered in colleges of veterinary medicine.

Veterinary Medical Doctor (VMD). The degree awarded to graduate veterinarians by the College of Veterinary Medicine at the University of Pennsylvania.

veterinary medical extension. That branch of veterinary medicine that provides animal health information to pet owners, farmers, and veterinarians, usually under the auspices of colleges of agriculture or veterinary medicine.

veterinary medicine. The profession that deals with the diagnosis, treatment, and prevention of animal diseases.

veterinary public health. The branch of veterinary medicine that deals with animal-borne human diseases.

veterinary technicians. Persons trained and qualified to work with animals under the direct supervision of a veterinarian.

Veterinary Services. An agency of the US Department of Agriculture that deals with a variety of animal health issues.

veterinary technology. The four-year college-level training program required of veterinary technologists.

veterinary technologists. Veterinary technicians with four years of college-level training, who work under the supervision of veterinarians.

virology. The study of viruses and the diseases they cause.

viruses. Microorganisms smaller than bacteria, which multiply only within the cells of living organisms.

VMCAS. See **Veterinary Medical College Application Service**.

West Nile disease. A mosquito-transmitted, often fatal, neurologic viral infection of horses, characterized by a variety of nervous disorders. It originated in Asia and Africa and is now present in the US.

Western equine encephalomyelitis (WEE). A mosquito-transmitted viral infection of horses and birds, present in western US and Canada and parts of South America and Central America. It also infects humans.

white muscle disease. A sometimes fatal muscular degeneration that occurs in calves and lambs due to deficiencies of selenium and vitamin E. It causes stiffness and sometimes recumbency. It is characterized by paleness and whitening of many muscles including those of the heart. It is preventable by injections of selenium and vitamin E. See also **stiff lamb disease**.

World Organisation for Animal Health (OIE). The world's oldest international animal health organization, headquartered in Paris and formerly called the Office International des Épizooties. When changing its name in 2006, it retained its original abbreviation (OIE).

yellow fever. An acute viral infection of humans, transmitted from nonhuman primates to people by mosquitoes, and characterized by fever, vomiting, and jaundice.

zoo animal medicine. The practice of veterinary medicine on zoo animals.

zoo animals. Wild animals, usually of nondomestic origins, kept in zoos.

zoonoses. Animal diseases that are transmissible to people.

zoonotic diseases. See **zoonoses**.

BIBLIOGRAPHY

1. Crawford, Jane D. 1995. *The Pre-Veterinary Planning Guide*. New York: Williams & Wilkins.
2. Kahan, C. M., Editor, 2005. *The Merck Veterinary Manual*. 57th Edition. Whitehouse Station, NJ: Merck & Co. Inc.
3. Kahrs, R. F. 2008. *Mastering Scientific Writing*. West Conshohocken, PA: Infinity Publishing.
4. Kahrs, R. F. 2009. *The Highway to Writing Success*. West Conshohocken, PA: Infinity Publishing.
5. Carnegie, Dale. 1998. *Dale Carnegie's Lifetime Plan for Success, How to Win Friends and Influence People* and *How to Stop Worrying and Start Living*. New York: Galahad Books.
6. Haynes, N. B. *Keeping Livestock Healthy*. 4th Edition. 2001. North Adams, MA: Storey Books.
7. American Veterinary Medical Association. 2008–2009. *AVMA Membership Directory & Resource Manual*. 57th Edition. Schaumburg, IL: American Veterinary Medical Association.
8. Prasse, K. W., Heider, L. E., and Maccabe, A. T. "Envisioning the Future of Veterinary Medicine: the Imperative for Change in Veterinary Education." Schaumburg, IL: *Journal of the American Veterinary Medical Association*: Vol. 231, No. 9. Nov. 1, 2007. 1340–1342.
9. Kahrs, R. F. 2003. *Viral Diseases of Cattle*. Ames, IA: Iowa State University Press, a Blackwell Publishing Company.
10. Kahrs, R. F. 2004. *Global Livestock Health Policy: Challenges, Opportunities, and Strategies for Effective Action*. Ames, IA: Iowa State University Press, a Blackwell Publishing Company.

About the Author

Bob Kahrs grew up on Long Island and attended Malverne High School, where he played football and basketball and ran on the track team. He spent his summers working on dairy farms in Connecticut, Pennsylvania, and upstate New York and spent one summer as a migrant farm worker. While still a veterinary student, he married his college sweetheart, Evelyn Payne. They have four children and six grandchildren.

After six years of college, he received the DVM degree from the New York State College of Veterinary Medicine at Cornell University and entered the veterinary profession.

He spent a year in a mixed practice in Interlaken, NY, and six years in his own practice in Attica, NY. He then spent 16 years teaching veterinary medicine at Cornell, where he served on the admission committee for eight years and served as its chairman for four years. While there, he learned the trials and tribulations of candidates for admission and the challenges facing admission committees.

In 1977 he became a department chairman at the University of Florida and gained new insights into the challenges facing veterinary medical education. In 1982 he became dean of the College of Veterinary Medicine at the University of Missouri and learned about university administration and politics.

After ten years at Missouri, he worked for the USDA for seven years, negotiating import and export requirements for animals and animal products. Later, he served as the part-time Coordinator of International Affairs for the Association of American Veterinary Medical Colleges.

Throughout his career, he was expected to write. Initially, he detested this chore. Because he had waded through ponderous manuscripts and textbooks in search of clear messages, he worked to achieve writing clarity and reader comfort, and eventually came to enjoy writing.

He has published *Viral Diseases of Cattle*[9] and *Global Livestock Health Policy.*[10] Later, to share his writing experience, he published *Mastering Scientific Writing*[3] and *The Highway to Writing Success.*[4]